Stopping

Scoliosis

Stopping Scoliosis

The Whole Family Guide
to Diagnosis and Treatment

2ND EDITION

Nancy Schommer

AVERY · A MEMBER OF PENGUIN PUTNAM INC. · NEW YORK

Every effort has been made to ensure that the information contained in this book is complete and accurate. However, neither the publisher nor the author is engaged in rendering professional advice or services to the individual reader. The ideas, procedures, and suggestions contained in this book are not intended as a substitute for consulting with your physician. All matters regarding health require medical supervision. Neither the author nor the publisher shall be liable or responsible for any loss, injury, or damage allegedly arising from any information or suggestion in this book. The opinions expressed in this book represent the personal views of the author and not of the publisher.

Most Avery books are available at special quantity discounts for bulk purchase for sales promotions, premiums, fund-raising, and educational needs. Special books or book excerpts also can be created to fit specific needs. For details, write Putnam Special Markets, 375 Hudson Street, New York, NY 10014.

AVERY

a member of
Penguin Putnam Inc.
375 Hudson Street
New York, NY 10014
www.penguinputnam.com

Library of Congress Cataloging-in-Publication Data

Schommer, Nancy.
Stopping scoliosis : the whole family guide to diagnosis and treatment /
Nancy Schommer.—2nd ed.
p.   cm.
Includes bibliographical references and index.
ISBN 1-58333-121-2
1. Scoliosis—Popular works.   I. Title.
RD771 .S3 S24   2002   2001053668
616.7'3—dc21

Printed in the United States of America
3   5   7   9   10   8   6   4

BOOK DESIGN BY MEIGHAN CAVANAUGH

This book is dedicated to the members of
the Scoliosis Research Society.

Acknowledgments

I wish to thank the following individuals and organizations (listed alphabetically) who assisted me in the preparation of *Stopping Scoliosis*:

The American Academy of Orthopaedic Surgeons; Fred Barge, D.C.; Ronald Blackman, M.D.; Oheneba Boachie-Adjei, M.D.; Thomas D. Borkevec, M.D., David Bradford, M.D.; William P. Bunnell, M.D.; Cynthia Clark-Shufflebarger, R.N.; Dennis Crandall, M.D.; Robert Dickson, M.D.; Joseph Dutkowsky, M.D.; John Emans, M.D.; Laura B. Gowen, L.H.D.; Serena S. Hu, M.D.; Vicki Kalen, M.D.; Hugo Keim, M.D.; Howard King, M.D.; Michael LaGrone, M.D.; John E. Lonstein, M.D.; Thomas G. Lowe, M.D.; Ronald Moskovich, M.D.; Alf Nachemson, M.D.; Clyde Nash, M.D.; The National Scoliosis Foundation; Michael Neuwirth, M.D.; Joe O'Brien; James Ogilvie, M.D.; Charles T. Price, M.D.; Linda Racine; Frank Rand, M.D.; Thomas Renshaw, M.D.; The Scoliosis Association; The Scoliosis Research Society; Joseph Sweere, D.C.; Robert Winter, M.D.; and Bettye Wright, P.A., R.N.

Special thanks to all the scoliosis patients and their parents who shared their experiences with me.

Contents

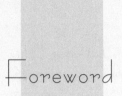

Foreword

When *Stopping Scoliosis* was first published, *Publishers Weekly* applauded the book as "a compassionate, informative guide to the diagnosis and treatment of curvature of the spine." *Kirkus Reviews* hailed it as "a concise, clear explanation of scoliosis and its treatments, with plenty of practical pointers and support from fellow sufferers." Those comments are as true now as they were then. I am pleased to have the opportunity to say that the new edition of Nancy Schommer's book is, in my opinion, the best, most comprehensive book currently available for the layperson who is dealing with this baffling disorder.

If you have been diagnosed as having scoliosis, you should find the answers you're looking for in this book. As she worked on this latest edition, Ms. Schommer interviewed many of the best-known orthopedic spinal specialists in the world to get the most up-to-date information available. With her gift for translating medical jargon into readable prose, she supplies readers with important, accurate information that is easily understood. What's more, because she has had two surgeries to correct her own scoliosis, she is able to write about her subject with sensitivity and compassion; she understands what it's like to wear a brace and to undergo surgery, and she shares her insights with candor, humor, and warmth.

Stopping Scoliosis is an invaluable resource for anyone dealing with this challenging, perplexing condition.

Laura B. Gowen, L.H.D.
Founder and President Emeritus
National Scoliosis Foundation

Stopping Scoliosis

Introduction

I see her every morning when I buy my cup of coffee at a bustling New York deli near my office. She darts back and forth behind the counter, quickly jotting down orders and stuffing bagels into white paper sacks. I watch her every move.

Perhaps seventeen, she reminds me of myself when I was that age: quick, birdlike movements; sarcastic, rapid-fire banter—and a petite, wiry body that is beginning to show signs of scoliosis.

She's just as clever as I was roughly thirty years ago, but she's invented her own special way of hiding it. The preppy-looking sweater draped about her shoulders provides near-perfect camouflage. So does the smock that billows over her uniform. But every time she bends to reach into the glass case filled with pastries, I can see that her body has begun to betray her. The gnarled spine gives away her secret.

I see her every morning and the same thoughts race through my mind. Surely she must know she has scoliosis—curvature of the spine. Surely she can't ignore that twisted torso, those uneven shoulders. Surely a parent or a friend has tried to coax her into seeing a doctor about it. Then it hits me: Maybe she's too proud—or scared—to admit that something's wrong. Maybe she's convinced herself that nothing can be done.

I'll probably never know the truth. I know I can't just walk up and confront her—she looks too cocky, too much like me, to accept that sort of approach. Maybe one of these days, when she's not so busy, I'll con her into having a cup of coffee with me so that I can at least tell her a story. Maybe parts of it will sound familiar to her.

Sweat trickled down the sides of my face as I spun the dial on the combination lock that secured my gym locker. As I fumbled to open it, the girl next to me pulled off one of her tennis shoes and slam-dunked it into the towel bin.

"That woman is a real sadist!" she shrieked. "Did you see who I got stuck with today? Jeez, what a pizza face!"

I chuckled, but knew just how she felt. This was the most dreaded semester in all of tenth grade—endless weeks of "modern dance," during which we spent an hour a day stumbling around the gym floor in the awkward grasp of pimply faced boys.

"Yeah, well, did you see my partner?" I asked. "He's only about a foot shorter than me, and I swear he kept trying to look down my shirt. What a creep! Thank God I had my bra on."

"Bra? You call that 'trainer' a bra?" she teased. "Face it, Schommer, you're a plank."

My breasts were in training all right, but I thought they showed a lot of promise. In no time at all, I figured, I'd be graduating to one with real cups—the push-up kind that were guaranteed to "lift and separate." All I needed was a little more time to grow. . . .

The locker room echoed with the hoots and hollers of my classmates as we got undressed and prepared to hit the showers. I quickly wriggled out of my gym suit, wrapped a tiny white towel around me, and—quite cleverly, I thought—managed to undo my bra with one hand, slide it down the front of my body, yank it out from beneath the towel, and toss it into my locker, all in one fast, fluid movement. I sat down on the bench, slipped out of my panties, and flicked them into my gym bag with one foot. We had all become masters of deception when it came to undressing in front of one another, but I felt I had the routine down to a science.

"Schommer, what on earth are you doing? What are you trying to hide?" My gym teacher's voice bounced off the wall behind me. I clutched my towel and crossed my legs as I watched her walk toward me. She was, with her short-cropped hair, squat neck, and thick legs, what we called a real jock.

"Get rid of that towel and get into the shower," she barked.

"What do you mean?" My voice squeaked out the words.

"You heard me. We do not take our towels into the shower. I told you that weeks ago. Honestly, you girls and your modesty! Now ditch that towel and start lathering up!"

Amid all the mumbling and grumbling—none of us liked the "no-towel" rule—I reluctantly dropped it, turned around, and tiptoed quickly across the cold granite floor, my arms flanked across my breasts. She was watching every move I made and seemed genuinely pleased at my embarrassment.

"Wait a minute, Schommer. Come back here."

I fully expected a loud lecture and imagined that the girls would crowd around me while the old crone held me up to ridicule. But instead she gently took my arm, led me to a secluded area beyond earshot of my classmates, and handed me a towel. Shivering, I grabbed it and held it close.

"Stand up straight for a moment, would you, Nancy?" Her voice was so soft and gentle I couldn't believe this was the same woman who, moments ago, had tried to make a fool of me.

"What do you mean?" I asked. "I am standing up straight." Her eyes narrowed to slits; she was studying every inch of my body.

"Would you mind turning your back to me?" she asked. Oh, come on, I thought, you're just trying to torment me. Can't you see this towel isn't big enough to cover my behind? Slowly I pivoted and faced the wall.

"Have you noticed anything different about your back lately?" she asked.

"Nope. Why? What do you see?"

She put her hands on my waist and pushed in on each side.

"Can you feel that?"

"Feel what? Your hands are cold." My heart was racing now.

"Let's go over to the mirror for a moment," she said as she led me toward the bathrooms. Gently she pulled the towel to one side. "Now, do you see how one hip looks higher than the other? Can you see that little indentation on the left side of your waist?"

"No, I don't see anything," I said, without really looking. "Can we just stop doing this now?"

"Okay. I'm sorry if I've embarrassed you. But I think you may have a slight curvature of the spine. That would account for your hips looking uneven. Have you ever seen a doctor about it?"

"I just had a complete physical and I checked out okay. My doctor's a really terrific guy. He'd have said something." Actually, it had been nearly a year since I'd had my last physical exam, but I wasn't up to quibbling about details. Besides, I felt just fine.

"Well, maybe it's nothing," she said. "But I think it's something you ought to watch."

"Yeah, I'll watch it," I said angrily. "I'll watch it every day and let you know what happens."

During the next several months, I did everything I could to avoid thinking about my spine. But all around me there were clues that pointed to one disturbing fact: my "slight curvature" was getting progressively worse. And so, one morning, I marched straight into the bathroom, locked the door, took off all my clothes, and stood directly in front of the full-length mirror.

Head up, shoulders back, feet planted firmly on the floor, I studied every contour and ripple. I rested my hands on my hips and pushed inward. Yes, there did seem to be a slight indentation on the left side of my waist. And yes, my right hip did seem to be tilted slightly higher than the left. But the difference was so minute, I had to keep looking again and again. One moment it seemed higher; the next it seemed level with the other one. Now I was getting confused. Was there really something wrong, or was I imagining things? Maybe the little dent marked the beginning of a womanly waistline. But then why wasn't there another one on the other side? And what about the hip? What would explain its asymmetry? My thoughts drifted back to the locker room. "Slight curvature of the *spine*," the gym teacher had said. As I scrutinized my body, her comment made no sense at all. What could a slight curvature of the spine have to do with my hips?

I shifted my weight from one foot to the other, watching carefully the effect this had on my body. When I raised my left foot off the floor, my hips leveled off. After a few minutes of repeating this little soft-shoe routine, the idea finally hit me: one leg was shorter than the other. That was the problem! But how to solve it?

Half an hour later I was sitting on the edge of the toilet seat, cutting thin pieces of cardboard into small heel-shaped discs. I stacked three of them in the heel of my left shoe and looked at myself in the mirror. No discernible change in my hips. I continued inserting cardboard pieces until they reached a quarter-inch thickness. Another glance in the mirror. I seemed level at last!

I practiced walking back and forth across the room, trying to adapt to my new shoe lift, but the only way I could keep the cardboard pieces from sliding around in my shoe was by shuffling. This would never do, I thought, so I glued them together into a solid piece. Now it was easy to walk around. Better than that, the little dent at my waist seemed to have disappeared!

As you might have guessed, this gambit didn't work. What with all my activities at school, I couldn't seem to keep the lift a secret—to my horror, it slipped out of my shoe onto the floor at least once a day. And when I removed it at night, my body returned to its slightly crooked position.

Mind you, I didn't look "deformed." But even though my hips would be facing straight ahead, the upper part of my body, particularly my rib cage, seemed to be curling slightly to the left. By this time I wasn't feeling any kind of pain; my earlier aches, probably caused by stress or my body's reaction to my first menstrual period, had all but disappeared. Now all I felt was vague discomfort, for which I could get relief only by repeatedly twisting myself back to the right.

Throughout my junior and senior years, I had the ominous feeling my body was fighting against some unseen force that was determined to keep me out of balance. Eventually, there was no denying it anymore. Something was wrong with my body, and I felt it had to be something more than a slight curvature of the spine. Something slight would not cause such gnarling. Whatever it was, I knew it was serious.

I was scared, but waited until after I graduated to make an appointment with a doctor. I figured if I'd gone this long, certainly a few more months couldn't hurt.

He poked at me, ran his fingers up and down my back, and told me that I had a spinal curvature. I was fully expecting that he'd prescribe a bunch of exercises, maybe even a new type of heel lift. Instead, he told me I'd have to wear a back brace for a year. That would keep the curve from getting worse, he said. And he assured me it wouldn't be nearly as bad as I thought.

The contraption I wore for the next twelve months was the closest thing to an eighteenth-century corset that I'd ever seen. It laced up the front, wound tightly around my body so that I could hardly breathe, and had two metal bars that jutted out from the back and stopped about an inch above my shoulder blades. At the top of these bars thick straps of nylon were attached; I'd pull them over my shoulders and attach them to little belt buckles that held them—and me—in place. Once rigged up, I felt I was in a straitjacket.

Unfortunately, this "back brace" (which I have since learned was intended for people suffering from low back pain, not scoliosis) did not fix my curvature. At the end of my year of confinement, at the age of eighteen, I was more gnarled than ever. I was also angry; I had spent a year looking like a freak, and for what? Now I looked worse! I kept my wrath to myself, though; I didn't have the guts to confront this man who, like many doctors in the 1960s, was probably unaware of, or at least unschooled in, the complex disorder known as scoliosis.

I didn't have to wait long to get my own firsthand lessons about the sinister spinal deformity called scoliosis. In fact, six months later, I heard the word officially for the first time, during a physical exam that was required by the University of Minnesota for all entering freshmen. The doctor took one look at me, asked me to bend over, then shook his head.

"Well, you certainly have scoliosis," he said, peering over the horn-rimmed glasses that perched on the end of his nose. "Why'd you wait so long to see a doctor?"

I was sure the doctor wouldn't want to hear the saga of how, despite all the clues I'd been given along the way, I chose to ignore my "slight" curvature of the spine. Besides, I just wanted to get on with it. What did it mean that I had scoliosis?

Before I got my answer, the doctor sent me to an on-campus orthopedic center that specialized in the diagnosis and treatment of the disorder. There I had a series of x-rays taken and met a scoliosis specialist. He, too, was nonplussed that I had blithely disregarded my curvature, which now twisted within my body at more than 40 degrees. But instead of blaming me, he addressed himself to the task of explaining scoliosis to me.

Unfortunately, his medical lexicon—words such as "lateral curvature," "vertebral rotation," "skeletal maturity," and "Cobb angle"—only served to baffle me. He did, however, utter one word that I had no trouble deciphering: "surgery."

I can think of no other moment in my life when I was as frightened or as dazed. In fact, I can hardly recall what the doctor and I talked about after he said the magic word. But that's where the haziness ends. My memories of the two spine surgeries I would eventually undergo to correct my scoliosis are as vivid as any I have tucked away.

Those surgeries, done for different reasons, were highly successful. Indeed, I have no regrets whatsoever about either surgery. Today, my posture is the envy of my peers. You wouldn't guess that I'd ever had anything wrong with my spine. But let's not let a little healthy body worship skew the facts. Because of ignorance, pride, and fear, my family and I allowed my scoliosis to reach a point where, over time, it required two surgeries— a grand total of eight hours on an operating table and sixteen months in a plaster body cast, plus untold hours of anxiety to straighten it out. Worse than all that, the entire ordeal probably could have been avoided!

1

What Is Scoliosis?

The more you know about scoliosis, and the sooner you know it, the more likely you are to stop it from progressing. If you've picked up this book because you think you have scoliosis—or know someone who may have it—you've taken the first important step toward conquering it.

Let's begin by taking a look at a normal spine and learning how, through the sometimes mysterious forces of nature, this marvelous architectural foundation of the human body follows a crooked path called scoliosis.

The Normal Spine

Of the more than two hundred bones that make up the entire human skeleton, perhaps the most gracefully shaped and intricately formed structure is the *spine*. Although people often like to refer to it as the *spinal column* or *backbone,* both of these terms can be misleading because they give the impression that we are speaking about one long, solid mass of bone. If that were true, you would never be able to nod your head up and down while saying "yes" when someone asked you for a date, nor could you shake your head from side to side when you pleaded, "No, honest, Officer, I wasn't speeding." Furthermore, you wouldn't be able to arch your back during an exam to get a little relief from tension, and it would be impossible for you to bend over and pet your dog. Indeed, if our spines were solid structures, we would go through life looking like rigidly constructed robots.

But thanks to the architectural talents of Mother Nature, our spines consist of approximately thirty-two individual bones in young children and twenty-six or more in adults, each slightly different, that are stacked one upon another, beginning at the top of the neck and ending in the neighborhood of the rump. Each of these bones is called a *vertebra* (derived from the Latin verb *vertere,* which means "to turn"), and several of these bones together are called *vertebrae.* The spine is sometimes referred to as the *vertebral column.*

Understanding the Vertebrae

If you run your fingers down the middle of your back, you'll feel a series of bumps or knobs. Each one represents one part of a single vertebra. Now imagine that you have removed one vertebra from this mid-back area and are holding it in your hand so that the bump you felt is closest to your wrist. This is the position represented in Figure 1.1, which gives you a clear "aerial" view, as if you were looking down through your body at an individual vertebra.

Most of your vertebrae, like the one pictured in Figure 1.1, have three bony protrusions. The one that you feel as you run your fingers down your back is called the *spinous process.* On each side of this bony structure is a *transverse* ("sideways") *process;* in the thoracic, or middle, area of your back, these protrusions connect to your ribs.

In the center of each vertebra is an opening called the *vertebral,* or *neural, canal.* It surrounds your spinal cord, which sends messages from your brain to all the other parts of your body and is protected by the bone of the spine.

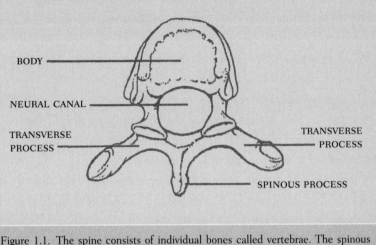

Figure 1.1. The spine consists of individual bones called vertebrae. The spinous process of this thoracic vertebra is one of the bumps you feel when you run your fingers down the middle of your back.

In front of the neural canal is the body of the vertebra—the solid, cylindrical element that most of us visualize when we think about the spine.

The Vertebral Groups

To understand more about how the spine is constructed, it is helpful to look at the various groups of vertebrae and to learn the special names of each one.

Imagine that you have drawn a horizontal line extending from the bottom of one earlobe to the other. At the center of this line, inside your skull, is the first of the seven *cervical vertebrae*. The word *cervical* derives from the Latin word *cervix,* meaning "neck." The uppermost vertebra is called the *atlas,* named after the giant in Greek mythology who held the heavens on his shoulders. Just beneath the atlas lies the second cervical vertebra; it is appropriately called the *axis,* because it is this vertebra that allows you to move your head in a twisting motion. Beneath these are stacked five more vertebrae. They don't have special names, but people in the medical profession often refer to them by numbered designations—as C3, C4, C5, and so on.

The next group is comprised of the *thoracic vertebrae*. The word *thoracic* comes from the Greek word thorax, which means "chest." Twelve in all, these important vertebrae not only give you support when you lean against the back of a chair, but are the structures to which your twelve pairs of ribs are attached. The thoracic vertebrae are commonly referred to by number—T1, T2, T3, and so on, through T12.

If you put your hands around your waistline and slide your thumbs toward the center of your back, you will be touching the first vertebra in the *lumbar* (from the Latin *lumbus,* meaning "loin") group. The five vertebrae in this area hold up the weight of most of your upper body. As a result, they are the largest vertebrae of the spinal column. Without the lumbar vertebrae, you would not be able to bend over. (See Figure 1.2.) Like the thoracic vertebrae, the lumbar vertebrae have numerical designations (L1 through L5).

Now move your hand to about the middle of your rump. What you'll feel is the *sacrum* (from the Latin word for "sacred"). At birth, this area is made up of five tiny vertebrae. As the body grows, however, they fuse together into a solid mass of bone. The sacrum, the hipbones (or pelvic girdle), and the coccyx are joined together to form the pelvis. The sacrum is the main support of this structure.

If you plop down on a chair, you'll be sitting on the triangular structure (made up of three tiny vertebrae, sometimes fused in adults) called the *coccyx,* the lowest portion of the spine. Sometimes referred to as the "tailbone," the coccyx is so named because it somewhat resembles the beak of a bird (in Latin, *coccyx* means "cuckoo").

The spine is far more than just an intricate structure made up of vertebrae. From the axis to the sacrum, each vertebra is connected to the next vertebra by ligaments and muscles designed to help us bend easily. In addition, wedged between each pair of adjacent vertebrae is a rubbery, cylindrical structure called an *intervertebral disc.* Made of fibrous tissue, or gristle, surrounding a pulpy nucleus, the discs absorb the shocks that occur each time we walk, jump, run, or bend in any number of directions.

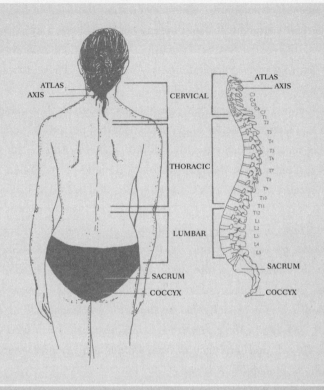

Figure 1.2 The vertebrae of the spine are named according to their position within in the body. For example, the bones in the neck are called cervical vertebrae; those in the lower back are called lumbar vertebrae. Named and numbered according to location, the first thoracic vertebra is referred as T1, the second T2, and so on.

The Shape of the Spine

When you look at a person with a normal spine, viewing him or her from the side, you see that even though the individual may have great posture, his or her back is anything but straight.

From the atlas to about the seventh cervical vertebra, the spine curves slightly forward, then slopes gently backward through the thoracic, or chest, area, then forward again in the lumbar area toward the sacrum. All normal spines have this gentle, S-shaped curve, but we are rarely aware of it, because a normal spine, when viewed from the front or back, appears to be perfectly straight. If the spine curves toward the front or back to an abnormal degree, the result, in the upper back, is called *kyphosis*—"round-back"—or, in the lower back, *lordosis*—"swayback." These, too, are spinal deformities, but they are not scoliosis.

If someone's spine begins to show signs of curving from side to side, known as a *lateral curve*, we begin to suspect that person has scoliosis. But does that mean that anyone with a side-to-side curvature of the spine has scoliosis? Consider the thought-provoking remarks of Dr. Robert Dickson, an orthopedist at St. James's University Hospital in Leeds, England:

> *If a scoliosis surgeon was presented with a spinal x-ray and a protractor [a device for measuring the size of a curve], he could probably find a scoliosis somewhere in the spine, albeit of small magnitude. There seems to be no inherent reason why a spine consisting of [many] vertebrae piled on top of each other, separated by gristle and held up by guy ropes, growing in three dimensions simultaneously for at least fifteen years in girls and seventeen in boys, should actually ever be straight, and in all probability, it is not.*

Perhaps, then, most of us have a "touch" of scoliosis. But what's important is how much of a touch do you have, how is it affecting your body, and will it get worse?

When a Curve Worsens

Although a side-to-side curve in the shape of a C or an S is the hallmark of the disorder, scoliosis is more complicated than that. In many cases, as the curve progresses—that is, increases or worsens—the spine also begins to rotate. It "curls" toward the hollow, or concave, side of the curve, and in advanced cases that affect the thoracic area, the ribs attached to the spine shift as well. The ribs on the concave side crowd together, while those on the convex side splay apart. (See Figure 1.3.) Eventually the entire rib cage may narrow and become egg-shaped, crowding the heart and lungs

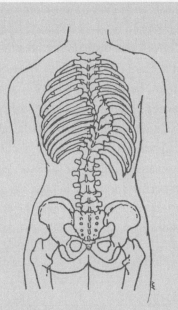

Figure 1.3. A scoliotic curve not only curves from side to side, but also rotates and causes the ribs to shift to an abnormal position. In advanced cases, rotation can cause problems in heart and/or lung function.

and choking cardiopulmonary functions. In rare cases, people with scoliosis can even die because their curves shut off their ability to breathe normally.

Idiopathic Scoliosis

Although scoliosis can be caused by a birth defect, a severe accident, aging and brittle bones, or neuromuscular disorders such as muscular dystrophy and polio, in 80 percent of all cases it occurs for no apparent reason at all. Hence doctors call these most common of all spinal curvatures *idiopathic,* a term used to refer to a disorder that has no known cause.

Idiopathic scoliosis can begin in any of three stages of life. When it occurs from birth to three years of age, it is called *infantile idiopathic scolio-*

sis. This type is usually found in boys. Considered a rare condition, the infantile curvature improves on its own without treatment in nearly 95 percent of all cases. Although scientists do not know why, infantile scoliosis is far more prevalent in Europe than in the United States.

When scoliosis strikes between the ages of four and ten, it is referred to as *early-onset idiopathic scoliosis* or, occasionally, as *juvenile scoliosis*. This type of curve occurs in both boys and girls, and can progress fairly rapidly as the child approaches adolescence.

The third type of scoliosis, and by far the most prevalent, is *adolescent idiopathic scoliosis*. It occurs during the adolescent growth spurt—usually between the ages of ten and thirteen—when the skeletal frame is developing most rapidly. For unknown reasons, it strikes girls in seven out of every ten cases.

What Causes Scoliosis?

I put that question to Dr. Alf Nachemson, professor of orthopedic surgery at Göteborg University in Sweden, who has surveyed the world literature on research into the causes of scoliosis. He scratched his head, smiled, took a very deep breath, and provided me with what he called a "mere sample" of causes—some more plausible than others—that have been proposed over the years:

Scoliosis patients have "crooked" mothers or "crooked" fathers, one leg is shorter than the other or one arm is longer than the other. The scoliosis patients grow too quickly and menstruate too early, they cannot look straight with their eyes, and they do not talk intelligently. They have poor postural stability, their spinal nerves do not grow enough, and their muscles show asymmetrical strength.

Heaving a sigh, he continued:

Their muscles contain abnormal fibers, as well as viruslike bodies. Their body chemistry has gone haywire. Their vitamin C intake is too small; their sugar intake is too big. They have strange elastin fibers everywhere. Platelet abnormalities are also found in their blood. Their discs grow in the wrong direction, their spines become unstable, and their joints stiffen up.

Finally, as the lines of his face relaxed, he said, "I shall stop here, but I could actually continue for a long time."

When you think about it, why should there be only one causal explanation for a disorder that can present itself as a C or S shape in nearly a dozen curve patterns, some with more vertebral rotation than others? And how could just one cause explain why, for example, two nearly identical young ladies, both with 30-degree curvatures, have completely different outcomes? One may go through life without her curve ever progressing another degree, while the other, even after wearing a brace for years, may eventually develop a curve of such magnitude that it can be treated surgically only.

Such diversity has led many orthopedists and scientists to conclude that idiopathic scoliosis may not be just one disorder after all. Says Dr. James Ogilvie, an orthopedic surgeon at the University of Minnesota:

Now we tend to lump most of these curves—C- and S-shaped, thoracolumbar patterns, and all the others, progressive and nonprogressive— into one category called "idiopathic scoliosis." But eventually, I think we're going to find that we're not dealing with the same disorder at all. In fact, I can't assure you that five to ten years from now we'll even be able to say that right and left curves are in the same category.

This phenomenon has occurred in medicine before. A hundred years ago, when researchers studied pneumonia, for example, they figured that whether people were coughing up blood or phlegm or fluid, they all had one disease called pneumonia. But now we know many different microbes can cause many different kinds of pneumonia and that they're really very different diseases. And by way of analogy, I think we'll find the same thing will be true of idiopathic scoliosis.

At the beginning of this new millennium, researchers are still trying to track down a logical reason why an otherwise perfectly healthy individual develops a spinal curvature. According to Dr. Thomas Lowe, clinical professor at the University of Colorado Health Sciences Center in Denver, "Although a large body of information about the deformity has been accumulated, we still don't know what the cause is, but the current trends in research may lead us to the answer." Those trends were outlined in the August 2000 issue of *The Journal of Bone and Joint Surgery* in an article written by Dr. Lowe and some of his colleagues who are members of the Scoliosis Research Society. Dr. Lowe summarized their findings as follows:

> *We know there is a genetic link—the prevalence is much higher among relatives of patients with scoliosis than in the general population—but we don't have the genetics figured out even closely yet. We do know that the prevalence of severe scoliosis is very low and that isn't changing. Some researchers are studying the role of hormones such as melatonin, which have an effect on the immune system and sleep patterns. Others are looking at calmodulin, a protein found in muscle and platelets, which regulates the function of muscles and may play a role in curve progression during the period of rapid growth. Studies have shown some differences in melatonin and calmodulin in patients with scoliosis related to asymmetry of the spinal musculature with indirect effects on growth mechanisms. A number of colleagues continue to pursue research in the areas of abnormalities of connective tissue, skeletal muscle, the spinal column, and the rib cage, but these are thought to be secondary to the deformity itself. Research also continues with respect to neurological abnormalities in patients with idiopathic scoliosis. Those involved in this work believe it is possible that a defect in processing by the central nervous system affects the growing spine. Despite all of our efforts, however, the true etiology [origin] of idiopathic scoliosis remains unknown. The best we can say at present is that it is a multifactorial disorder.*

Who Develops Idiopathic Scoliosis?

Unfortunately, doctors cannot yet predict with great certainty who among us will get idiopathic scoliosis. But if you ask orthopedists just how many youngsters in the United States are likely to develop a lateral curvature, you usually get this answer: 1 in every 50. That sounds like a lot—until you realize that not all curves are serious or require treatment.

According to Dr. John Lonstein, an orthopedic surgeon at the Twin Cities Spine Center in Minneapolis, Minnesota, and one of the researchers who keeps track of the percentage of the population afflicted with scoliosis, the best way to understand the prevalence of the disorder is to convert that estimate of 1 in every 50 by using proportionately higher figures. Thus, we may say that 20 out of every 1,000 youngsters will develop a lateral curvature. "Out of these 20," says Dr. Lonstein, "15 youngsters will develop curves of less than 20 degrees—degrees are a measure of the amount of curvature in the spine—but few of these will get worse. The remaining 5 of every 1,000 will have curves greater than 20 degrees, but on average, only 1 or 2 of these will increase and require treatment."

Can You Be Born with Scoliosis?

The answer to this question is yes. This condition is known as *congenital scoliosis*. It is far less common than the idiopathic variety. In these cases, says Dr. Ronald Moskovich, an orthopedic surgeon affiliated with the Hospital for Joint Diseases in New York City, "the vertebrae did not form properly during fetal development and they are therefore not the normal rectangular shape we expect to see. Indeed, a variety of vertebral abnormalities can cause the spine to curve. For example, half a vertebra may be missing, which we call a hemivertebra; the resulting wedge-shaped vertebra tilts the spine over in one direction. Sometimes, two or more vertebrae are joined together on one side or the other; they haven't separated as they should in utero and this basically blocks the proper growth of the spine." Although these conditions are sporadic and rare, and the incidence of congenital scoliosis is a fraction of a percent compared with that of the idiopathic variety, Dr. Moskovich notes that "you can get progressions of 6 to 10 degrees a year, which is huge. So if the curve measured 10 to 20 degrees at birth, it could increase to 50 to 60 degrees within a few years." Many varieties of congenital scoliosis, however, are mild and may not progress with growth. Careful monitoring and recognition of the various scoliosis patterns is key to deciding how and what to treat.

In general, congenital scoliosis does not respond to brace treatment. The reason? There is a physical abnormality in the bone itself, not just in the alignment of the spine. Therefore, in those cases in which treatment is required, surgery is the only option.

It is important to note that individuals who have congenital scoliosis often have congenital abnormalities in some other part of their bodies as well. About a third of them have kidney or bladder abnormalities, and roughly twenty percent of those who have congenital scoliosis of the cervical spine also have hearing problems. Some also have heart conditions.

Types of Spinal Curves

Doctors have identified nearly a dozen different curve patterns in scoliosis. However, for our purposes, we will look at four major types of curves that can occur: the right thoracic, thoracolumbar, lumbar, and double major curves.

RIGHT THORACIC CURVE

The *right thoracic curve,* which centers itself in the chest area, is the most common of all. It usually starts at the T4, T5, or T6 thoracic vertebra and ends around T11, T12, or L1, the first lumbar vertebra. (See Figure 1.4.) Such a curve can progress rapidly and, unless treated early enough, will shift the ribs on the right, or convex, side and create a deformity that's known as a *rib hump* on the back. Not only is the hump unsightly and the

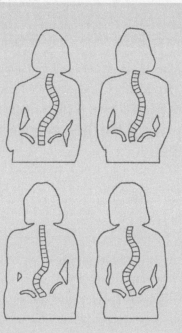

Figure 1.4. Although doctors have identified nearly a dozen curve patterns, the most common types of curve are: right thoracic (*top left*); thoracolumbar (*top right*); lumbar (*bottom left*); and double major (*bottom right*).

cause of much psychological stress for the person who has developed it, but it is also dangerous, because it can squeeze the heart and lungs, causing serious cardiopulmonary problems.

THORACOLUMBAR CURVE

The *thoracolumbar curve,* which begins in the chest area at T4, T5, or T6 and ends in the lower back at L2, L3, or L4, may twist to either the right or the left. (See Figure 1.4.) Although it is less deforming than a right thoracic curve, the thoracolumbar type usually creates an asymmetrical torso.

Lumbar Curve

The *lumbar curve* occurs in the lower back and appears at T11 or T12 to L5. (See Figure 1.4.) In roughly 65 percent of all cases, these curves shift to the left. A lumbar curve will twist the hips so that they appear uneven and can cause a great deal of back pain, particularly in adults and especially in pregnant women.

Double Major Curve

The *double major curve* is the most prevalent of the S-shaped curves that occur with scoliosis. The upper part of the curve occurs in the thoracic or chest area, while the lower part affects the lumbar area. (See Figure 1.4.) Because one curve offsets the other, the double major curve is considered more balanced and less deforming than the single C-shaped curves. But if it becomes severe, it can cause a rib hump.

How Scoliotic Curves Are Measured

If methods for measuring curves hadn't been devised, doctors would have a hard time distinguishing between mild, moderate, and severe curves. And how confusing it would be to learn that you have a "really big" curve or a "pretty small" one! Thanks to the late Dr. John Cobb, an orthopedic surgeon with the Hospital for Special Surgery in New York City, who developed one of the most successful methods for measuring curves, doctors now describe scoliotic curves in terms of degrees.

To measure an S-shaped double major curve, your doctor would begin by taking an x-ray of your spine. Then he or she would start measuring the top curve, using a straightedge to draw one horizontal line just beneath the highest vertebra involved in the curve, and another just above the lowest curving vertebra. From these your doctor would draw perpendicular lines that eventually intersect to form an angle. That angle would be measured and referred to in degrees. The doctor would then repeat these steps to measure the bottom curve. (See Figure 1.5.)

Because scoliotic curves often rotate, as well as curving from side to side, doctors have developed a method for measuring the amount of spinal rotation. As you can see in Figure 1.6, a line is drawn on an x-ray in the center of each vertebra involved in the curve. If rotation is present, the oval indentations (called *pedicles*) on each vertebra shift progressively closer to the midline. To describe the relative proximity of the pedicles to the midline, doctors will refer, for example, to a +1, +2, +3, or +4 rotation.

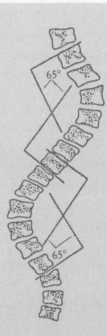

Figure 1.5. To determine how many degrees a spine is curving, most doctors use the Cobb angle of measurement. Each curve of this double major curve has a Cobb angle of 65 degrees.

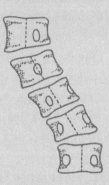

Figure 1.6. If rotation is present in a curvature, the pedicles (oval indentations) on each vertebra appear closer to the midline that the doctor draws on the x-ray.

Whose Curves Must Be Treated?

Let's say that you suspect you have scoliosis. You meet with an orthopedist who believes it is necessary to take x-rays of your spine. After the doctor measures the Cobb angle of your curve, then figures out how much, if any, your spine is rotating, he makes this pronouncement: "You have a right thoracic curve of 22 degrees, +1 rotation." Okay, now you know without a doubt that you have scoliosis. Your next question is, "What should I do about it?" To your utter surprise, the orthopedist replies, "Well, you may not have to do anything at all."

Nothing? Do nothing about the curve? Don't I have to wear a brace or have surgery?

The answer to these questions depends, in part, upon the maturity of your bones, or *bone age*. Girls usually stop growing at about age sixteen. Boys, a little slower in the growth department, reach maturity at around age eighteen. But since we all grow at slightly different rates, these dates may vary. Thus, a girl who is chronologically fourteen may have already reached maturity, whereas a boy of eighteen may still be skeletally immature.

How Bone Age is Determined

To determine your bone age, your doctor may go back to that initial x-ray and examine the *iliac crests* of your hips. You can feel these on either side of your body by placing your hands just beneath your waistline. In people who are skeletally immature, these crests appear to be separated from the rest of the bony pelvic girdle; in those who are skeletally mature, they have fused together into a solid piece of bone.

Individual vertebrae also can provide clues to bone age. In immature youngsters, the *growth plates* that are located at the top and bottom of each vertebra have not united with the vertebra. When maturation is complete, these plates (seen on an x-ray) appear to be fused to each vertebra.

Your orthopedist may also take an x-ray of your hand and compare it to scores of other hand x-rays that have been catalogued in a book called the *Atlas of Greulich & Pyle.* Such a comparison might reveal that a girl who is chronologically fourteen actually has a bone age of thirteen.

Dr. James Ogilvie of the University of Minnesota explains it this way:

If you take a young lady who is twelve years old with a 22-degree curvature, and she's been menstruating for two years, and is wearing a bra, and has shapely hips, you may say she's only twelve calendar years old, but when you look at her bones on x-rays and see that the growth centers have all closed, you'd say she had a bone age of fifteen or sixteen. She would have already gone through the growth spurt, and we'd consider her skeletally mature. We'd continue to watch her curve, but it's unlikely that it would progress. She might not have to do a thing about her curve.

But if you took another young lady of twelve with a 22-degree curvature, and she hadn't started menstruating yet and didn't have what we call secondary sex characteristics, we'd say this child is in a high-risk group to have a progressive curve. We'd watch her carefully, and if her curve progressed, we'd begin treatment immediately.

Prognosis and Treatment

Predicting which curves will worsen is a laborious and often difficult task for orthopedists. But because they have amassed so much information about curves over the years, they can provide us with a few general guidelines. For example, most experts now agree that slight curves—between 10 and 15 degrees—are hardly worth worrying about, as long as they don't progress. Still, people do fret about them, according to Dr. Ogilvie:

> We frequently see people who've been told by their doctors that they have scoliosis and they come to our clinic with red lights flashing and a 12-degree scoliosis, which means absolutely nothing. Not only can it not be cured, it does not need to be cured. It's like having someone come in and say, "My doctor told me I have red hair! What do I do about it?" We don't worry about such small curves if they're not progressing—they do not have, as we doctors say, prognostic significance, which is another way of saying they're not the kinds of curves we treat.

Depending on the bone age of a person and the location and size of the curve, when it progresses to within a range of 20 to 40 degrees, doctors usually recommend that the person wear some sort of brace designed to stop the curve from progressing. But this rule of thumb holds true only for adolescents whose bones are still growing. Curves in adults cannot be stopped or improved by braces.

If a youngster's curve progresses beyond 40 degrees, the best solution is surgery. "For adolescent curves of that magnitude," says Dr. Ogilvie, "surgery is the only way to stop the curve. With adults, we'd evaluate a 40-degree or greater curve on a case-by-case basis. Some adults can live with a curve of that magnitude. Others cannot, because their curves deform them, or interfere with their heart and lungs. In these cases, we can perform surgery, often with excellent results. But if people paid a visit to a scoliosis specialist at an earlier age, in most cases, surgery could be avoided."

Early detection—that's the key to preventing and arresting a curve caused by idiopathic scoliosis. But there always will be individuals whose curvatures go unnoticed. Some kids learn to compensate for their condition (often without even realizing it); they look normal and participate in activities just like anyone else. Many slip past the scoliosis screening room because there is no way to enforce screening in our schools. And there will always be adults who, because they are too ashamed of the way they look or because they are convinced nothing can be done for them, will continue to suffer needlessly from their scoliosis.

Whether you are an adolescent or an adult with scoliosis, you should know this: There are treatments available today that can stop your curve from progressing and surgical techniques that can transform a gnarled body into one that's a delight to the eye. But to find out whether you can benefit from these treatments, you must first figure out whether you have scoliosis. As you will see in the next chapter, there are special ways of detecting the disorder—diagnostic techniques that can help save you, or someone you love, from a lifetime of deformity and pain.

2

Keeping the Odds in Your Favor

How important is early detection and treatment of scoliosis? Perhaps no one knows better than Dave Elmore of Jasper, Indiana, an astonishingly courageous man (now in his fifties) who spent the better part of his life battling against a spinal curvature that reached an astounding 134 degrees. "It robbed me of twenty years of my life," he says, "stripped me of self-confidence, warped my attitude toward life—all because nothing was done about it early enough."

Although there is a bright side to Dave's story—after enduring several surgical procedures to correct his scoliosis, he is in relatively good health today—you cannot ignore the fact that he, as he puts it, "paid heavy dues to get there." Indeed, if you asked him about the importance of early detection, he'd sit you down, look you straight in the eye—"not caring whether or not you could see that I still have a slight hump"—and take you back to 1959, when his troubles began:

I was fourteen or fifteen back then, and my mom noticed that I wasn't standing straight. She thought I was slouching a lot of the time. To be honest with you, I never noticed that there was anything wrong with my back. I don't ever recall thinking, "Gee, my back is curved." But Mom sensed something was wrong, so she hustled me to a local physician, who did x-rays, and there it was—a curvature of about 35 degrees. He said, "Dave, there's nothing we can do for you. The bones have set in place, a brace is out of the question, and we can't operate on you. Wear loose-fitting clothing. If there's pain, take some aspirin. Mostly, just be thankful you're alive. It could be worse." He also told me that the curve would stay right where it was—it wouldn't get better, but it wouldn't get any worse.

I took his word as gospel. I mean, he was a Doctor with a capital D, right? So I just figured I'd have to live with it, that nothing could be done for me.

That guy was dead wrong about my curve not getting any worse. As it progressed, I developed a hump on my back that I couldn't ignore— I'd wake up every morning and see the hump! And there was no hiding it, either. If I'd go into a clothing store and pick out a suit I liked, it would have to be altered, or else one leg would end up being longer than the other. I couldn't even wear an ordinary pair of Levi's. I'd walk down the street and hear people saying, "Hey, look at that guy." As a result, I became very self-conscious and introverted. I knew I was different physically, and became more and more shy. Maybe that's just part of the male ego—you want to be like the other guys, but you know you're not and it bugs you. So I dealt with it by hiding from society for twenty years!

I had a lot of pain and it just kept on getting worse. Have you ever had someone take a pliers to your skin and pull it? That's what it felt like sometimes. It's almost like there was something in my back trying to get out. I tried everything I could think of to kill the pain. I did a lot of sleeping on the floor, and in a two-week period I took a hundred aspirin.

Because of the pain, I lost a lot of time from work, which didn't exactly please my employer. At one point he demanded that I bring him a doctor's excuse to explain a recent absence. That, believe it or not, was how this body finally got into the right hands.

An acquaintance whose wife had had scoliosis surgery suggested I see her doctor. So off I went, figuring I'd hear the same song and dance: "Sorry, Dave, there's nothing we can do for you."

What the doctors said to me was almost worse than that: My scoliosis, now at 134 degrees, was killing me! It was twisting my body and squeezing my heart and lungs. My heart was enlarged, and my right lung was so deformed that my breathing capacity was about half of what it should be. That came as news to me—I hardly ever paid any attention to the fact that I was short of breath most of the time.

I could hardly believe that all that was happening to my body. But what surprised me more was this: the doctors said they could do something about it!

I trusted them immediately, although I know I'd have trusted the devil if he'd said something could be done. I especially liked the fact that they sat me down and explained the facts to me—they didn't sugarcoat them or beat around the bush about the risks involved. And there were plenty of risks. The surgery was going to be tricky because some of my vertebrae and ribs had grown together. I had the beginnings of arthritis as well. But mostly they were worried about the danger of respiratory failure during the operation—they said my body and organs might have trouble coping as they straightened my spine.

The doctors said I'd probably be in the hospital for three to six weeks and have to have maybe two or three surgical procedures performed on me, plus I'd be in a cast for perhaps six months. But it didn't turn out quite that way.

Between January 3 and March 18 of 1983 I was in the operating room six times, and they performed seven separate surgical procedures on me. I was in the hospital for nearly two and a half months and in bed so long that it got to the point where I'd forgotten what a floor felt like!

The doctors took me apart, physically and mentally, and put me back together again. And it was a pretty hairy roller-coaster ride all the way. I was scared a lot of the time, one of my legs was partially paralyzed, and I had about every complication you can think of. But all things considered, I'd do it all again. I don't remember ever feeling this good! I just wish I'd had it done a lot earlier."

Back then, all of Dave's surgeries combined—including hospitalization and surgeons' fees—cost in excess of $37,000. That seems like a lot—and it is—until you consider that today, just one single-stage surgery (including hospitalization and fees) can cost in the upper ranges of $35,000! And a two-stage, anterior-posterior procedure—becoming more popular all the time—can run from $70,000 to $85,000 or more.

You'd think that these astronomical figures would convince all state legislatures to require public schools to screen for scoliosis in about the fifth grade. Unfortunately, only twenty-two states have done so to date: Alabama, Arkansas, California, Connecticut, Delaware, Florida, Georgia, Indiana, Kentucky, Maine, Maryland, Massachusetts, Nevada, New Hampshire, New Jersey, New York (except for New York City, Buffalo, and Rochester), Pennsylvania, Rhode Island, Texas, Utah, Vermont, and Washington.

Curves Still Go Undetected

Even if you live in one of the states that has recognized the importance of early detection of scoliosis, there's a chance that your scoliosis, or that of a family member or friend, could go undetected. There are several reasons for this:

- According to Dr. John Lonstein, orthopedic spine surgeon with the Twin Cities Spine Center in Minneapolis: "In today's schools, screening for scoliosis has a low priority. Nurses have less time and money than ever before, so the time spent on screening is way down. Furthermore, nobody checks to see who's being screened and who isn't, and there's no penalty if it's not done."
- Many youngsters whose bodies are just beginning to develop are self-conscious and will go out of their way to avoid being seen in the nude.
- A person who has scoliosis can "compensate" for a curve or conceal it by deliberately raising a crooked shoulder or wearing bloused clothes. I know this firsthand: By the time I had made the decision

to have surgery, many of my friends and coworkers were shocked to learn there was anything wrong with me. "Why on earth are you having surgery?" they asked. "We can't tell you have a curvature of the spine!"

- There are certain kinds of curves that are less noticeable than others. According to University of Minnesota orthopedic surgeon James Ogilvie: "If you have just a single C-shaped thoracic curve, which tends to be more cosmetically devastating than an S-shaped curve, and it reached 70 degrees, you'd look crooked. Yet someone with an S curve—70 degrees right thoracic and 70 degrees left lumbar—might not look bad at all. Even a parent wouldn't be able to see much wrong. And some people happen to have more rotation to their vertebrae than others. You could find two people who both have 50-degree curves—one has a lot of rotation, which causes a very sharp rib hump and cosmetically is just awful, whereas the other person doesn't have much rotation, and, to the untrained eye, you can't tell the curve is there."

If you think you or a family member has scoliosis, there's no reason why the curve should go undetected. There are a number of techniques available that can even help people with no medical background whatsoever to spot a curve before it's too late.

What to Look For

Let's say you have a fourteen-year-old friend who slumps a lot and sometimes seems to be leaning to one side. Hardly a day goes by that her parents aren't reminding her to "stand up straight!" When she wears a dress or a skirt, her hemline often appears crooked, leading you to believe that perhaps her parents are right—there is something wrong with her posture. But is her problem really poor posture? Or is it scoliosis?

To find out, you need to get a clear view of your friend's body, which means she should remove all clothing except her underpants. If her hair is long, she should pin it up so that her neck is in clear view. She should then stand with her back toward you. Her feet should be planted firmly on the floor to ensure proper balance, and her arms should hang loosely by her sides. Ask her to hold her head up in a comfortable position and to look straight ahead.

Now look at her overall posture. (See Figure 2.1.) If it's normal, you would be able to draw an imaginary straight line from the center of her head to the middle of her buttocks. Her shoulders would be level, and her shoulder blades would be symmetrical as well as being equal in prominence. Her hips would also be level and symmetrical, and there would be an equal distance between her arms and body. If your friend's body matches this description, it's a safe bet her problem is posture, because she is able to straighten herself up by standing properly. But if she has sco-

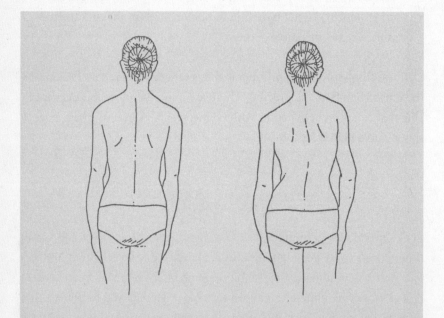

Figure 2.1. In a person with a normal spine (*left*), the head is in line with the buttocks; the shoulders and hips are level and symmetrical. Scoliosis may exist (*right*) if the shoulders and hips are uneven and the waist appears creased on one side.

liosis, her curvature will be apparent in one or more ways even when she's standing straight.

You might, for instance, see any number of clues that point to a curvature of the spine. If you draw that imaginary vertical line from head to buttocks on a person who has scoliosis, the line won't match up with either; the head seems to be shifted off to one side of the buttocks. You may also notice that one shoulder seems higher than the other and that the shoulder blades are uneven—one shoulder blade may appear to be jutting out farther than the other. As you look at her hips, you may notice that one side looks bigger or more prominent than the other, and you may see a crease at the waistline on one side or the other—that's the little "dent" that plagued me. Moreover, the distance between her arms and her body may appear to be unequal.

In addition to examining your friend while she's standing up straight, you should watch her body carefully as she performs what is called the *forward bending test*. This test is part of the screening examination used in schools across the country and can help you identify a scoliotic curve.

For this exam, ask your friend to put her hands together, palms and fingers touching, and bend forward at the waist with her head down. She should be standing with her back toward you. If her spine is normal, you will notice that both sides of her upper and lower back are symmetrical and that her hips are level and even.

If she has a spinal curvature, you may instead see that her rib cage and/or her lower back are asymmetrical. Sometimes this unevenness appears as a hump located about the shoulder or the lower back. (See Figure 2.2.)

Now ask your friend to face toward you as she bends at the waist with her hands held together as before. If her spine is normal, this front view will reveal that both sides of her upper and lower back are symmetrical. If not, you'll see an unequal symmetry of her upper back or lower back, or both. (See Figure 2.3.)

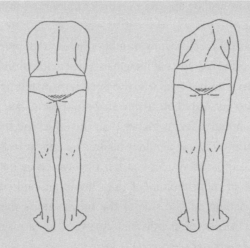

Figure 2.2. Viewed from the rear in a forward bending test, the normal spine (*left*) shows both sides of the upper and lower back as symmetrical and the hips as level and even. Scoliosis may exist (*right*) if the rib cage and/or lower back are asymmetrical, with the unevenness appearing as a hump.

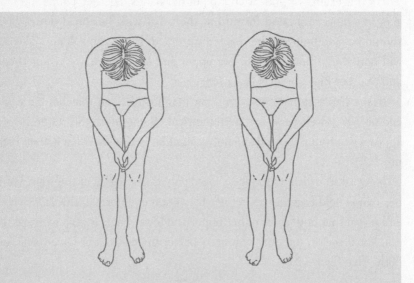

Figure 2.3. Viewed from the front in a forward bending test, the normal spine (*left*) shows both sides of the upper and lower back as symmetrical. Scoliosis may exist (*right*) if the upper back appears as asymmetrical or humped.

Is Pain a Symptom of Scoliosis?

The answer to this question depends on whom you ask. In the course of my research, I have talked with many youngsters with scoliosis who claim they *did* have discomfort before they were treated with a brace or with surgery. Typical complaints are occasional numbness or tingling in the legs, aching in one or more areas of the spine, and sharp pain about the neck and shoulders. In later life, adults with scoliosis can experience a great deal of pain, particularly because of breathing problems, ruptured discs, or arthritic conditions that can develop because of scoliosis.

But what do doctors say about pain and its role in adolescent idiopathic scoliosis? Here's a typical sampling of responses:

- "If a youngster with a spinal curvature complains about pain, we would look for some other cause of her curvature—a tumor or a disc perhaps. If there's pain in a youngster, it's probably not idiopathic scoliosis."
  —DR. JOHN LONSTEIN, ORTHOPEDIC SPINE SURGEON, TWIN CITIES SPINE CENTER, MINNEAPOLIS, MINNESOTA

- "I always ask my patients about this and at least a third tell me they have some mild discomfort, such as muscle soreness around the apex of curve. Typically, the pain is quite mild, and it is not what sent them to the doctor. There seems to be some muscle fatigue sort of phenomenon—it's not just "all in their head."
  —DR. VICKI KALEN, PEDIATRIC ORTHOPEDIC SURGEON, KERNAN HOSPITAL AND THE UNIVERSITY OF MARYLAND, BALTIMORE

- "As a general rule, we consider scoliosis to be a pain-free condition. However, there is evidence that in some individuals, mild, aching discomfort may well be related to their scoliosis. The aching may be muscular, or may have to do with the joints being loaded asymmetrically—nobody knows for sure."
  —DR. HOWARD KING, ORTHOPEDIC SPINE SURGEON, INTERMOUNTAIN ORTHOPAEDICS, BOISE, IDAHO

- "When all these attractive kids—fourteen, sixteen, eighteen, twenty years old—come in for operations, I always ask them why they want it done. They say, 'I hurt and I want it done.' If I press them a bit and ask them why again, they'll say, 'Because it's getting worse and it bothers me. I'm active in sports and everything, but my clothes don't fit and it really hurts.' After we do the operation, when I ask them how they feel, the first thing they say is, 'Well, how do I look?' If I were a patient with scoliosis, I'd want that deformity fixed. And if I thought the doctor wasn't going to operate because he's not a cosmetic surgeon, he's just going to operate if there are structural problems and pain, I'd tell him it hurt, because I'd want the thing fixed."
  —DR. DAVID BRADFORD, ORTHOPEDIC SPINE SURGEON, UNIVERSITY OF CALIFORNIA, SAN FRANCISCO

Whether it's real or imagined, pain alone is not a reliable indicator of scoliosis. And even though the standing and forward bending tests are quite effective in helping reveal a spinal curvature, they are merely tools of detection. They cannot tell you whether or not a curve will progress, nor can they ensure that you get the proper treatment. Only a trained scoliosis specialist can make educated guesses about whether a curve will get worse and whether you can benefit from the many breakthroughs in non-surgical and surgical treatment that are available today.

Monitoring Your Curve

If a screening exam reveals a spinal curvature, it doesn't mean you need to be treated immediately. Most often, particularly if a curve is mild, a doctor will prefer to watch it for a while to see whether it progresses.

In many areas of the country, a series of x-rays, taken every four to six months or so, is used to monitor a curve. Depending upon the nature and location of your curve, you may have to have as many as four x-rays per visit—standing (front and back), supine (lying down), and bending from side to side.

X-Rays — and What You Need to Know about Them

Upon hearing that multiple x-rays may be required to monitor a curvature, many people become worried that they will receive "too much" radiation; they fear that their bodies will be penetrated by doses large enough to alter or destroy bodily tissue. Are these fears warranted? To find out, I interviewed Dr. Joseph Dutkowsky, an orthopedist at the University of Virginia. This is what he told me about x-rays:

Q: *Who discovered x-rays?*

A: The German physicist Wilhelm K. Roentgen (pronounced *rent-gen*) discovered them in 1895. During one of his experiments, he noticed that radiation not only penetrated through the skin so he could see deeper structures like bone tissues, but it also produced phosphorescence, or light. Because he didn't really know what these mysterious rays were, he named them "X" rays. Today, we know that this kind of radiation is all around us—in the atmosphere, in the ground beneath our feet, and even in our own bodies. We're all radioactive. And it has nothing to do with what we eat or drink—it's just the way we're put together.

Q: *How much radiation is produced by a scoliosis x-ray compared with other sources of radiation?*

A: The standard unit of radiation is called a *rad*. For measurement purposes, we usually divide a rad into thousandths, which we call *millirads*. In other words, one-thousandth of a rad is one millirad. Now, to put that into perspective, consider a few figures:

- If you stayed outdoors all year round in New York City, you'd get 90 millirads of radiation.
- If you stayed in a brick building twenty-four hours a day for a year in New York City, you'd get 140 millirads.

- If you live outside the fence of a nuclear power plant, the United States government would allow you to get 125 milli-rads per quarter, or 500 millirads per year.
- If you have a dental x-ray, you'd get 1,000 millirads.

If a young girl has a scoliosis x-ray exam consisting of one posterior-anterior (PA, or back-to-front) x-ray, plus one lateral (side-view) x-ray, and assuming preventive measures have been taken to protect her breasts, her breast tissue would receive a total of 10 millirads.

Q: *How does one prevent overexposure to x-rays?*

A: The first preventive measure is to avoid x-radiation whenever possible. For example, during the course of treatment, a doctor may use a Scoliometer or other nonimaging method to monitor a patient's curve. [More about the Scoliometer and a nonimaging technique called moiré topography later in this chapter.] Unfortunately, though, devices like the Scoliometer cannot give us *exact* information about a curvature; only an x-ray can provide us with an extremely accurate picture of a curvature. And in certain instances—when a patient is seen for the first time and shows signs of scoliosis, or later on if his or her curve has progressed—a doctor may need to x-ray the patient in order to determine the precise nature and degree of the curve.

Q: *When an x-ray cannot be avoided, what do doctors do to lessen a patient's exposure to radiation?*

A: In the past several years, doctors have increased and standardized the distance of the patient from the x-ray machine. Patients now stand six feet from the machine, which automatically cuts down x-radiation exposure. Second, they've reversed the position of the patient who must have standing x-rays. Instead of having patients face the machine, which allows x-radiation to enter sensitive breast tissue first, we now turn them around so that their backs face the machine. This way, the spine and ribs absorb the radiation before it reaches the breasts.

Q: *What else can be done?*

A: Doctors use a variety of lead shields that block roughly 99 percent of the radiation generated via an x-ray machine. For young girls, whose breast tissue is the most sensitive to radiation, we use breast shields. Made of lead and covered with heavy cloth, they look a lot like aprons and cover the breast area during x-radiation. When necessary, we also use lead shields that protect a female's pelvic region, where the reproductive organs are located. For young boys, we use lead shields for the genital area. In addition, all modern x-ray machines have lead shields built right into them. By using the lead aprons for breasts and/or genitals, you're adding another measure of safety. At scoliosis clinics, using these aprons is a standard procedure. Scoliosis clinics also use devices called *rare-earth screens.*

Q: *What are rare-earth screens, and what do they do?*

A: Placed on each side of an x-ray film, rare-earth screens allow more light to flash on the film to expose it. Because rare-earth screens produce more light, you can use fewer x-rays to get the same picture. For that reason, all scoliosis clinics today use them.

Q: *What about the long-term risk of breast cancer for young girls who have had scoliosis x-ray exams?*

A: In 1979, Dr. Clyde Nash did a study indicating that the typical female adolescent with scoliosis would undergo twenty-two x-ray exams during the course of treatment. Due to those x-rays, he estimated the risk of breast cancer would increase 110 percent. In my most recent study, which takes into account the many preventive measures that I've already mentioned, we've found that the risk has been lowered to roughly one-quarter of one percent. In other words, assuming that twenty-two radi-

ographic examinations are performed over the course of scoliosis treatment—a far greater number of x-rays than one would
receive today—our findings reveal that the increased relative
risk of breast cancer is roughly two breast cancers per million
women examined. That's an extremely small number considering that the risk of a woman getting breast cancer in her lifetime in the United States is one in eleven.

Q: *Do you have any other recommendations for people who get x-rays?*
A: When you have to have an x-ray, ask questions about the equipment and procedures. Remember, you have the right to demand
any or all of the preventive measures mentioned above. The
patient's body is ultimately his or her responsibility. The more
you know about the care you're getting, the more informed and
comfortable you'll be—and that helps doctors do their jobs.

OTHER TECHNIQUES FOR MONITORING CURVES

Some orthopedists, such as Dr. John Emans, Director of the Division of
Spine Surgery at Children's Hospital and Professor of Orthopedic Surgery
at Harvard Medical School, are trying to lessen their patients' exposure to
radiation by using a technique called *moiré topography*. With this technique, the patient stands behind an illuminated, fine-lined grid that
throws a symmetrical pattern of shadows onto the contours of the back. If
the patient has scoliosis, the pattern is asymmetrical. Dr. Emans and others who use moiré topography record these patterns with Polaroid pictures
and compare photographs taken during successive visits to detect any
changes. "We're able to see pretty clearly when a curve has progressed,"
says Dr. Emans, "and patients don't have to worry about radiation
exposure."

Doctors also use a device called a Scoliometer to monitor curves. Developed by Dr. William P. Bunnell, Professor of Orthopedic Surgery at
Loma Linda University School of Medicine and pediatric orthopedic
and scoliosis surgeon at Loma Linda University Medical Center in Cali-

fornia, it is used primarily to measure the angle of rotation. It is thin and rectangular-shaped, about the size of a small envelope. A U-shaped glass tube filled with fluid has a small ball positioned in the center of it. When the doctor places this device on the back of a patient who is bending over, the ball quickly seeks the lowest point in the tube, from which the angle of rotation can be measured. The Scoliometer is also considered the "gold standard" for school screening programs. It has been used all over the world for that purpose.

Even though the Scoliometer and moiré topography are effective ways of monitoring curves, orthopedists must still rely upon x-rays to determine the exact nature and extent of a curve.

How Long Should Monitoring Continue?

The answer to this question depends on skeletal maturity. If a youngster has a mild curve and is still growing, the doctor may want to schedule a return to the clinic for observation in four to eight months depending on the maturity of the child and the size of the curve. Adults with moderate curves may not need to be checked for several years. According to Dr. John Lonstein, "The only adults we monitor regularly are those who have very large curves. And if the curve eventually stabilizes, monitoring would no longer be necessary."

In between visits to a specialist, young people with scoliosis (and their parents) can take an active role in the monitoring process. Watch for any changes in the size of your curve, the prominence of your ribs, your posture, and your height. Keep a written record (or take photographs) to document any signs of progression, and contact your orthopedist if you feel there is cause for concern.

Pregnancy and Scoliosis

In the past, many doctors believed that pregnancy would increase the risk of progression of a curve—as much as 6 to 8 degrees with each pregnancy—in a woman with scoliosis after she reached skeletal maturity. Of course, that was worrisome to women with scoliosis who wanted to have children—they assumed that because they had the disorder, they would have to forego the joys of motherhood or risk worsening the condition. But according to Dr. Bunnell, developer of the Scoliometer, scoliotic women who wish to have children have little to fear.

Referring to a study he did while he was at the Alfred I. duPont Institute in Wilmington, Delaware, Dr. Bunnell says:

> It was our early conclusive finding that pregnancy does not increase the risk of problems developing in patients with scoliosis. In other words, there is no increased risk that the curve will increase. In addition, there did not seem to be an increased incidence of back pain in the patients we studied. We also looked at the impact that scoliosis might have on pregnancy and delivery. Here, too, we found no increased incidence or problems including the need for a cesarean section, or any increased problems with the children. In essence, our findings show that women should be able to look forward to normal pregnancy and delivery with no increased risk either to themselves or to their pregnancy as a result of having scoliosis.

Curves Can Worsen in Adulthood

According to Dr. Hugo Keim, former chief of the spine clinics at the New York Orthopaedic Hospital of the Columbia-Presbyterian Medical Center in New York City (now retired), the worst advice a physician can give a patient with scoliosis is, "As soon as you finishing growing, your curve will stop."

Although orthopedists cannot predict whose curves will worsen in adulthood, Dr. Keim suggests that scoliosis is most likely to progress during adult life in the following groups of individuals: "Those with a strong genetic 'dose' of scoliosis; those with a curve pattern that throws the trunk out of balance, such as the thoracic, thoracolumbar, or lumbar curves; and those with extremely poor muscle tone, especially women who have become overweight and underexercised. Naturally not all scoliosis patients get worse as they get older, but curves in those who meet the previous criteria generally progress one to two degrees with each year of adult life."

Unless you are monitored by a specialist who knows that scoliosis can progress in adulthood, you run the risk of being told that you shouldn't be too concerned about your curve and that all will be well for the rest of your life. The remarks may be comforting at the time, but imagine how you will feel if your curve follows the same path as these patients of Dr. Keim:

A. D. was first examined for scoliosis at age thirteen years and three months. She then had a right thoracic curve of 33 degrees from T4 to L1. A well-meaning physician advised her that this was a mild curve and told her "not to worry" about it since it would "never get worse."

By age fifteen years and eight months her curve had increased to 45 degrees, but the advice was still the same. An orthopedist was consulted and also advised no treatment. This advice at first seemed correct because at age seventeen years and nine months the curve was still 45 degrees and seemed stable.

However, over the next nine years she noticed gradual curve progression and increasing back pain. When I met her, she was twenty-six years and eight months old and had a 61-degree curve. She noted shortness of breath during swimming and tennis and had curtailed these activities. Feeling so much more deformed, she experienced depression, had a poor social life, and believed she had been given the wrong medical advice by her previous physicians.

V. P., a twenty-one-year-old woman, had a left thoracolumbar scoliosis from T10 to L3. She was obviously fully mature and was told "not to worry" about her 20-degree curve. At age forty-two the curve had progressed only 5 degrees, and she was pleased that she had no pain. She had not married and had never been pregnant.

At age fifty-three the curve had progressed to 48 degrees (a 28-degree increase since age twenty-one), and she was beginning to have severe back pain and disability. She also had to give up her job as a beauty parlor operator. Surgery at that time had to be more extensive and complicated than preventive treatment at a younger age would have been.

M. K., a very attractive young lady, was under "observation" by an or-thopedist from age fourteen to twenty-eight. She had been told that her severe curves would not get worse because at age sixteen and a half she was "fully mature." She had a right thoracic scoliosis of 90 degrees from T5 to T11 and a left lumbar curve of 87 degrees from T11 to L4.

She was so concerned about health problems that she became a nurse and was examined on several occasions by orthopedists, who told her to "leave well enough alone." By age twenty-seven her right thoracic curve had increased to 105 degrees and the left lumbar curve also mea-sured 105 degrees. She was having marked shortness of breath and in-creasing back pain.

On her own volition, she sought surgical help for her curves and had successful surgery performed with satisfactory correction—for her age.

M. G., a twenty-six-year-old librarian, was first concerned about her scoliosis at age fourteen. Her curve measured 43 degrees. She saw sev-eral orthopedists over the next six years but was told that no further pro-gression would occur. At age twenty-six she appeared for treatment with a curve that measured 63 degrees. She was saddened and disillusioned by the poor advice she had received. A good surgical correction was ob-tained at that time, but not as much as she could have had at age sev-enteen when her spine was more flexible and the curve less severe.

Can Exercise Help?

Not only should you be wary of the physician who tells you "not to worry" about your curve because it won't progress into adulthood, you should also be suspicious of the doctor who recommends exercise as the sole treat-ment for your curvature. Any physician who does is misinformed, says Dr. James Ogilvie of the University of Minnesota:

Voluntary exercise alone will never improve or eliminate a curve, be-cause the brain cannot command specific paraspinal muscles [the mus-cles next to the spine] to contract and relax. It is those muscles and surrounding tissues, when strong and healthy, that keep a spine in a straight position. When they're weak on one side or the other, the spine will bend. And even if the brain could make the right connection, who would have the discipline or stamina necessary to carry out such an exercise program?

Although there are physicians who prescribe exercises for patients with scoliosis and who believe that daily exercise can help a curvature, none of them can provide concrete evidence that exercise is an effective solution to the problem of scoliosis. "There is no real scientific evidence that exercise will affect a curve that is progressing," says Dr. Lonstein. "When studies have been done on this, where half the kids are put through really intense exercises and the other half do nothing, there's no difference between the two groups. Although we know that exercise programs are quite popular in Europe, where kids are exercising for one to two hours each day, we don't yet know whether it's making any difference. So far, there's never been any documentation of results."

Until such data exist, scoliosis specialists will continue to try to spread the word that exercise is not a cure for scoliosis. The message needs to reach adolescents and their parents, as well as the medical students and residents who will become the specialists of tomorrow. Even though you would think these highly trained individuals would get the message through the medical grapevine, often they don't, which is why there are still many physicians prescribing exercises for their scoliosis patients. Thus, experienced orthopedists like Dr. Hugo Keim have tried to make the point perfectly clear in medical textbooks such as *The Adolescent Spine*. In this reference book, he makes an extremely persuasive case against exercise. Although it is intended to be read by physicians, this will give you a good deal of "insider" information about why exercises alone should be avoided:

One fact has been clearly shown . . . exercises never "correct scoliosis." They maintain and enhance body tone and are of value to the patient and family because they make the parents feel that they are doing something, which assuages their guilt feelings somewhat. However, do not be deluded that curve improvement could possibly be due to an hour or two of exercise which the patient may have done daily during the previous few months. The scoliotic spine is genetically programmed much like a computer to develop a specific curvature as growth progresses. This programming is determined by the genetic dose of scoliosis . . . received the moment the egg and sperm became one. The scoliotic curve that the patient will have [many] years hence can only be modified at specific times in the patient's life by either spinal bracing . . . surgery, or a combination of treatments. . . . Sometimes we see curves vacillate back and forth until the patient is fully mature with the final end result of a very mild curve. If an exercise program had been given to these patients, there would be hundreds of enthusiastic patients and parents who would gladly sign affidavits that exercises "did the trick."

Unfortunately, we cannot yet predict which scoliosis patients will improve spontaneously and which will get worse. We need a simple test which could tell us how strong a genetic dose of scoliosis a patient has inherited. We could then advise the family that the patient will never get worse or conversely that the patient has an extremely severe form of scoliosis and should be treated in the most aggressive manner.

To sum up the indications for an exercise program, you can prescribe it if you wish, as long as you understand that exercises only treat the psyches of the parents and help the muscle coordination of certain poorly muscled children, who are overweight and underexercised.

If your doctor prescribes exercises for you, make sure that he or she is doing it to help you improve muscle tone. If the doctor tells you that exercises alone will stop your curve, consult with another orthopedist immediately.

What About Chiropractic?

Unlike people with arthritis, for example, individuals with scoliosis have not yet been widely exposed to fraudulent treatments that claim to "cure" the disorder. You won't find splashy advertisements in the supermarket tabloids touting snake oil as a panacea for scoliosis, nor will you hear rumors that a few bee stings can stop a curve. But there is a branch of the medical community involved in scoliosis care that has become the focus of much controversy, and the pivotal question of the debate is this: Can chiropractic treatment prevent or stop a curve from progressing?

As you have probably guessed, the answer you receive depends upon whom you ask. According to one highly respected orthopedist, who asked to remain anonymous, but whose attitude reflects the opinion of many scoliosis specialists I interviewed:

> We've got lots of patients who come to us from chiropractors because they've gotten nothing out of manipulation. They come to us with curves that have progressed. Still, many chiropractors contend that they can help kids with scoliosis, and they offer us "proof"—in the form of x-rays, not scientific documentation—that they've done so. I can see why they think they're successful at treating scoliosis, because if they treat a hundred kids with manipulation, they're going to be "successful" with eighty out of a hundred, because eighty out of a hundred kids are not progressive anyway. In other words, if you do chiropractic manipulation on somebody who doesn't need treatment, you're going to get a fantastic result. Therefore some chiropractors believe they can help scoliosis. But some know they cannot.

Fred Barge, D.C., of the Barge Chiropractic Clinic in La Crosse, Wisconsin, is one of many chiropractors who believes that by adjusting the spine—using the hands to apply a thrust that repositions misaligned vertebrae—he can indeed correct a scoliotic curvature of the spine. Of course, Dr. Barge knows that these "dynamic thrusts" cannot benefit everyone with scoliosis, and he readily admits that "chiropractic never claims to cure any disease." Yet, based on his work with scoliosis patients throughout a career that spans forty-three years, he is quite convinced that "we can reduce curves if we get to them in time."

According to Dr. Barge, when vertebrae become "subluxated"—a term used by chiropractors to describe a misalignment—the center of the discs between these vertebrae shift to one side. "Like a teeter-totter," he explains, "the fulcrum shifts and causes what we call vertebral locking. The body responds to this by forming a scoliosis, and so my job is to help free up that locking, to restore the vertebrae to their normal position." When he applies those hand thrusts (adjustments) to the patient's back over a period of time, he says, "we can achieve an improvement."

Just how often a person needs these spinal readjustments is, in Dr. Barge's opinion, "determined by the amount of benefit the person is receiving. If a young girl came to me with a curvature under 30 degrees, and she was still growing, I might have her come in for adjustments twice a week for two months, then once a week for another month. Then I'd x-ray her again to see whether I was making any improvement, and if so, I'd continue caring for the child once a week for perhaps another four to five months. I'd reevaluate her again, have her come in every other week for a year, and when I'd achieved enough improvement, I'd recommend she make appointments monthly and receive adjustments when necessary."

When a patient's curve does not respond to chiropractic care, Dr. Barge often refers the individual to a scoliosis specialist: "One such patient was a girl of twelve. She was at the peak of her growth spurt, wearing a brace, and her curve was 58 degrees and progressing. She came to me and cried, saying she couldn't stand the brace, so I worked with her and tried to adjust her, but the curve just kept on getting worse. I was able to reduce her lumbar curve a bit, but the thoracic curve not one iota. I referred her to an orthopedic surgeon who corrected her thoracic scoliosis through the surgical implantation of rods. In her case, neither a brace nor chiropractic care could help."

Despite his willingness to refer highly curved patients to specialists, Dr. Barge says he is "not willing to go along with the opinion of many orthopedists that a curve cared for chiropractically would have gotten better by itself. Although we don't have any controlled studies to prove it, you can see the results spontaneously and objectively to prove our work."

Not all chiropractors share Dr. Barge's enthusiasm. In fact, according to Dr. Joseph Sweere, director of the Department of Occupational and Community Health at the Northwestern College of Chiropractic in Bloomington, Minnesota, "In an advanced case of scoliosis—and even a 20-

degree curvature is in my opinion a significant distortion—there's little I could do to make it better."

For Dr. Sweere and other chiropractors across the country who share his view, "the primary service of a chiropractor to the children of America is early evaluation and detection of a curvature. Often, by the time scoliosis is diagnosed, it's rather late to be seeing a chiropractor. Unfortunately, because we chiropractors are often the second, third, or fourth choice in terms of doctoring, we often get patients whose curves are quite advanced. We're considered the doctors of last resort."

Although Dr. Sweere believes such patients should be referred immediately to a scoliosis specialist, he does not rule out the possibility that a chiropractor might be able to help as well. But in such cases the person would probably seek the services of a chiropractor for relief of pain.

"I've never known of a better system to help pain," he says. "It simply works, and, for pain, chiropractic can be profoundly useful for those with scoliosis. If a lady is forty years old and having a backache due to a curvature, she certainly needs a good surgical opinion and workup—from more than one person—but there may be justification for a chiropractor to treat her as well. It may be the only relief this woman can get. In fact, I've had people come to me with 65-degree curves, and I send them to the scoliosis clinic for evaluation, where the doctors say to them, 'If you can get relief from a chiropractor, then do it.' Very often orthopedists will encourage their patients to see chiropractors for pain simply because it's a practical measure. But these are orthopedists who are open-minded—they're willing to work with us to aid a common cause."

Of course, that common cause should be the early detection and prevention of scoliosis. But until chiropractors can supply us with documented, scientific evidence that spinal manipulation really can treat curvatures, their primary function should be, as Dr. Sweere and others believe, in the area of diagnosis. "What's important to know about chiropractors," says Dr. Sweere, "is that they will probably continue to be criticized for not having controlled studies and will therefore continue to lack credibility in the medical community. It should be noted, however, that we lack controlled research studies because our profession, historically, has never had any financial support with which to do the studies it so desperately wants to do. Despite the criticism, however, chiropractors are licensed and obligated to diagnose scoliosis. Many chiropractors have had special training in orthopedics and, as such, can be trusted to do it well. They know what they can and cannot do for scoliosis. Others may not have the interest or inclination to deal with this rather complex problem. If there is any question as to the qualification of the chiropractor you have consulted, it is well to contact the Board of Chiropractic Examiners in the state in which you live."

Since it's unlikely that chiropractors will amass much scientific evidence about their craft in the near future, it's probably safer to rely on the treatments for scoliosis, discussed in the following chapters, that are currently available.

3

Nonsurgical Treatments

*For Children and Adolescents Whose Curves
Range from 20 to 40 Degrees*

Although people who have curves smaller than 20 degrees sometimes require treatment, the question of whether or not to brace or perform surgery arises most often in cases in which curves fall in the 20- to 40-degree range. (Once the spinal deviation approaches or exceeds the 50-degree point, studies show that skeletally immature patients' curves *will* progress into adulthood.) Doctors make recommendations for bracing or surgery based on a number of factors, including the size of the curvature, its location, and the skeletal maturity of the patient. This chapter surveys the major types of nonsurgical intervention prescribed for adolescents with scoliosis.

Rigid Bracing

Ever since the Greek physician Hippocrates (ca. 460–377 B.C.E.) began studying *skoliosis* (meaning "crooked"), doctors have tried to straighten the curved spines of their patients by using treatments that involve the application of forces to stretch and/or push the curving vertebrae. In most cases—at least until the twentieth century—their patients probably felt that the "treatment" was worse than having the disorder.

If you had lived centuries ago, your doctor might have strapped you to a medieval-looking rack for many hours at a time over a period of several months. Your arms and legs would have been forcibly stretched in opposite directions with an intricate system of weights, pulleys, and ropes. Or, because your physician figured that gravity played some part in pulling your spine and making your curve bigger, he might have opted for a "passive" cure—complete bed rest, for two or three years!

In time, doctors took a more sensible approach to caring for their patients; they tried to devise ways to straighten spines that would enable their patients to get up and move around. For some physicians, this meant bandaging a patient's body to splints—a rather cumbersome and uncomfortable way to keep a curvature from progressing. By the mid-1500s, treatments were much more sophisticated; with the help of armorers, doctors fashioned metal corsets that were intended to hold the body straight. But these "iron maidens" probably weighed twenty to thirty pounds. Under that kind of stress, patients no doubt ended up with rounded backs in addition to having scoliosis. These iron corsets eventually were replaced by ones made out of strips of leather, or by an innovative "jacket" that was molded from plaster of Paris.

Such plaster jackets represented the *haute couture* of braces at that time. They were relatively lightweight, were cheaper to make than the metal molds, and fit snugly to the body. It is also likely that they were more successful than their predecessors, if only because the people wearing them couldn't take them off. Of course, these plaster molds interfered with bathing and restricted the normal movements of the poor souls who were encased in them—especially those patients whose doctors, believing that more plaster meant more correction, kept on adding plaster until it covered the patient's neck and most of the head!

These plaster torture chambers provided passive correction; the brace did all the work to hold the body straight, and all the patient had to do was endure it. But some doctors believed their patients might do better with so-called active braces—devices that forced the body to interact with the brace.

In the late 1800s, physicians created a corsetlike contraption that bound the lower body in leathery material while metal bars that looked like suspenders fit over the chest and shoulders. Attached to these bars was a metal neck ring with sharp protruding buttons that fit just beneath the chin and behind the back of the neck. Unless the individual stood perfectly straight—indeed, he or she was forced to stretch and elongate his or her body—those irksome little buttons would jab fiercely into his or her skin. Needless to say, this brace was not very popular and probably did more harm than good.

Only within the last forty years have doctors developed rigid bracing techniques that are acceptable to the people who have to wear them. Most of the credit for this goes to two men: Dr. Walter Blount and Dr. Albert Schmidt of the Medical College of Wisconsin and Milwaukee's Children's Hospital. The brace they created is known, not surprisingly, as the Milwaukee brace. Although other braces are becoming more popular with doctors and patients alike, the Milwaukee brace is still the standard by which all other braces for scoliosis are judged. Most important, according to orthopedic spine surgeon John Lonstein of the Twin Cities Spine Center in Minneapolis, Minnesota, rigid braces, including the Milwaukee, can stop curves 80 to 85 percent of the time. Depending on where you live, a rigid brace can range from $1,400 to $2,000 or more. This cost should be covered by insurance. Let us look in more detail at some of the types of rigid braces available today.

THE MILWAUKEE BRACE

Although the Milwaukee brace was once considered the gold standard of braces for scoliosis, today it is used primarily for patients with kyphosis. (See page 14.) The largest component of the brace is a molded plastic pelvic girdle, to which a central bar is attached. From that bar, a strap winds around the body and is affixed to one of two metal bars in back of the brace. Depending on the specific type of curvature being treated, a brace may contain more than one of these straps, which hold specially designed pads that support the spine in the best alignment.

At the back of the brace, two metal bars run lengthwise and parallel over the shoulder blades. These bars rise to the back of the neck, where they converge with a throat mold, a sturdy piece of metal that encircles the neck like a collar or a ring. The pressure pads that push on the curve are attached to the sides of the posterior metal bars. The counteracting forces of all the pressure pads, the pelvic girdle, the neck ring, and an axillary sling (if required) hold the body straight. (See Figure 3.1.)

Even though the Milwaukee has the best and longest track record of all braces, it is cumbersome and uncomfortable, which is why people often resist using it conscientiously. Therefore, if your curvature is *not* in the high thoracic area of the spine, your doctor may prescribe a low-profile brace.

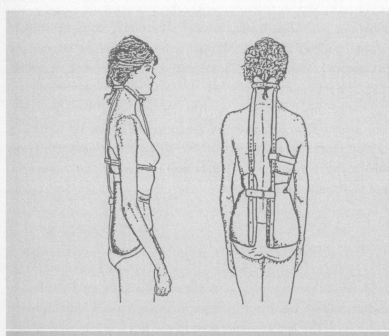

Figure 3.1. The Milwaukee brace consists of a pelvic girdle, throat mold, and various bars, straps, and pressure pads that work together to hold a curvature—that is, to try to prevent it from progressing further.

THE LOW-PROFILE BRACE

If you have a low curve, you will probably be able to wear an underarm brace called the *thoracic-lumbar-sacral orthosis,* or TLSO. This device is also known as an underarm brace or a Boston brace, after the city where it was developed by Dr. John Hall and Bill Miller in the 1970s. But depending upon where you live, you may get a similar brace with a different name—the Miami, the Wilmington, or the New York low-profile brace. (See Figure 3.2.) In Europe, similar braces are named the Ponte, Lyon, or the Riviera.

No matter what you call it, this type of rigid brace is extremely popular because it is not as bulky as the Milwaukee. The TLSO begins just beneath your armpits and under the breasts and ends near the pelvic area in the front and in the middle of your buttocks in the back. It is made of plas-

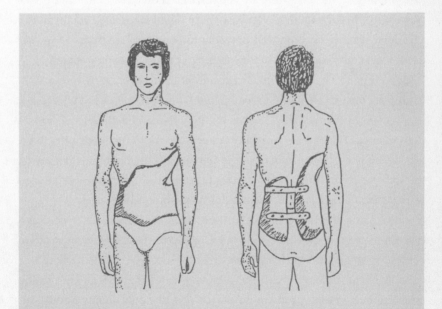

Figure 3.2. The low-profile brace is usually worn by patients with thoracolumbar and lumbar curves.

tic—either prefabricated or custom-molded—and is generally used on lumbar curves and some double curves. It may open in the front or in the rear. The TLSO also uses various types of pads to exert pressure on one side of the curve, while the brace itself (often molded a bit higher on one side) creates the counterpressure necessary to keep your body straight.

NIGHTTIME BRACING

At present, two types of nighttime braces are being tried in many parts of the country—the Charleston bending brace, developed by Frederick E. Reed, Jr., M.D., C. Ralph Hooper, Jr., C.P.O., and Charles T. Price, M.D., Chief of Pediatric Orthopedics and Surgeon in Chief at Nemours Children's Clinic, Orlando, Florida; and the Providence brace, developed by Barry M. McCoy, C.P.O., and Charles D'Amato, M.D., and colleagues. Both are similar to a low-profile underarm TLSO, except that they attempt to "overcorrect" the curvature by keeping the individual bent toward the convexity of his or her curve. Because these rigid braces keep you in an exaggerated leaning position that prevents most normal actitivies, they are used while you sleep (eight to nine hours per night is recommended).

According to Dr. Price, the Charleston brace uses bending forces—"It loads the convex side while unloading the concave side of the curve," he says—while the Providence pushes on the curve and provides traction in the same way that a TLSO or Milwaukee does. Both braces require plaster casting of the torso to make an initial mold. The mold and an x-ray of the spine are then sent to a fabricating plant, where computers help to determine the correct location of bending or pushing forces.

The Charleston brace has been used since the 1980s. Dr. Price says that there is good evidence that the Charleston works as well as other braces for single curves that are less than 35 degrees, particularly thoracolumbar and lumbar curves. For a curve greater than 35 degrees or for double curves, however, it would not be the brace of choice unless the physician and bracemaker have considerable experience with the Charleston brace.

According to Dr. D'Amato, "The Providence brace is effective for single and double curves under 35° and with an apex below the eighth thoracic vertebra. This has been validated in a study to be published in *Spine,* September 15, 2001."

Nighttime versus Full-Time Bracing

According to Dr. John Emans, a spine specialist at Children's Hospital in Boston, currently available data suggest that bracing of adolescent idiopathic scoliosis is probably "dose-related" and that for larger curves, full-time bracing (twenty to twenty-four hours a day until growth is completed) is probably more effective. In fact, he notes, a recent study undertaken at Texas Scottish Rite Hospital (TSRH) provides compelling evidence of this fact. "For consecutive periods," says Dr. Emans, "the center (at TSRH) used only full-time Boston TLSO bracing and then only Charleston nighttime bracing. All patients were followed for two years after brace completion. Although the nighttime-only brace was comparable with a full-time brace for milder curves, for moderate and more severe curves, full-time bracing appeared substantially more effective. Other centers throughout the country have also found the full-time brace more effective than nighttime bracing."

Certainly the choice between nighttime-only and full-time bracing is complex and multifactorial. Dr. Emans has concluded that, if possible, curves over 35 degrees—and in particular larger double curves—are probably better treated with full-time bracing. Nighttime bracing, on the other hand, is probably a better choice for adolescents with smaller curves who require bracing, particularly if the bracing is initiated early and the curve is a single lumbar or thoracolumbar curve. "Bearing in mind that the effects of bracing are dose-related," he says, "nighttime-only bracing is also the clear choice for the patient who refuses to wear the brace during the day."

Electronic Bracing

In the late 1980s, electronic bracing, also known as electrosurface stimulation, was considered by some orthopedists to be an alternative to rigid bracing. This technique involves using a hand-sized device that sends mild electric currents through the skin via electrode pads placed on the back over certain muscles. Early clinical trials showed that electronic bracing might stop some adolescent curves from progressing roughly 80 percent of the time. What's more, most patients actually *liked* using stimulators; all you had to do was use it every night until one's bones reached maturity, and the little transmitter did the rest. No daytime brace was required.

Since that time, however, this "wonder" device has fallen out of favor. Why? According to Dr. Thomas Renshaw, a professor of orthopedic surgery at Yale University in Connecticut, electrical stimulation has been unequivocally shown by every reputable study to be no better than no treatment at all. Just why it doesn't work, nobody really knows.

Dynamic Bracing

In the late 1990s, a promising new alternative to standard bracing became available. Developed by Dr. Christine Coillard and Dr. Charles Rivard, pediatric surgeons from Sainte-Justine Hospital in Montreal, the SpineCor bracing method provides flexible, inconspicuous correction that continues as a child or teenager moves and grows. The SpineCor brace consists of four elements: a plastic pelvic base; a cotton bolero or vest; tie bands; and four adjustable, or "dynamic," bands. The brace should be worn during the day and may be worn for up to twenty hours at a time. Depending on the individual's growth, follow-up visits may be needed every three to six months to make adjustments to the elastic bands.

According to Biorthex, Inc., the manufacturer of this device, it provides best results for individuals who are skeletally immature and have Cobb-angle curvature of less than 30 degrees. What do doctors think? Dr. Howard King, an orthopedic spine surgeon in Boise, who has prescribed the SpineCor for several of his patients, says that the early research data is promising, and that patients like it because it's like wearing an undergarment that is extremely flexible. In his opinion, it may be another option to bracing, and is worth looking into, but, he cautions, it is still in the early trial stages.

Getting Used to Your Brace

Most youngsters, when faced with having to wear a brace, have the same question: "How in the world will I ever get used to wearing this thing?" Many hope that their doctors will "wean" them into it a few hours at a time until their bodies and minds can get used to it. Alas, there is no weaning period. Once your orthotist has adjusted the brace so that it fits you perfectly, on it goes, for a period of time to be specified by your doctor. Some people must wear it daily for twenty to twenty-four hours, while others can still get good correction by wearing it twenty hours a day or less. Braces like the Charleston are worn primarily when you sleep.

Admittedly, the first few days are the worst. You think you'll never be able to tolerate the pelvic girdle squeezing your hips. If you're wearing the underarm type, you'll feel the back of it rub against your shoulder blades, while the bottom portion chafes against your hips and buttocks. If you're wearing a Milwaukee, it will seem as if that pesky neck ring always gets in your way, no matter which way you turn. Lean forward, and it pinches your chin; lean back, and those two pads seem to fight you every inch of the way. As for all of those metal bars—well, no matter if you're sitting, standing, or lying down, you feel as if you're being jabbed from every direction. And no matter which type of brace they're wearing, most young people can't imagine ever getting used to standing up *that straight!* You will get used to it, though. As your skin toughens, you'll no longer notice the rubbing and chafing, and any redness will eventually disappear.

What to Wear Under the Brace

The best way to counteract rubbing and chafing is to wear a T-shirt, leotard, or body stocking beneath your brace. (Girls can continue to wear a bra.) Make sure it fits snugly—excess material causes wrinkles, which will press in on your skin—and that it's seamless. Of course, you can adapt your undergarment to your needs—some kids who wear the underarm brace opt for wearing a tube top that can be pulled down snugly over the hips. If you have a Milwaukee brace, you can trim the arms off a T-shirt, if you like, and snip off excess material around the bottom near the buttocks so that the material doesn't bunch up beneath your slacks.

It's a good idea to pick an undergarment that's made of a natural fabric, such as cotton. It will breathe and allow excess perspiration to evaporate. Synthetic fabrics, such as nylon or polyester, tend to keep moisture trapped next to the body. Not only will such fabrics make you feel clammy, but the buildup of moisture against your skin will soften it and make it more susceptible to sores caused by rubbing.

Many brace wearers prefer to wear undergarments that have been tailormade for them. Constructed of soft cotton-blend material and considered by many to be more attractive than standard T-shirts, these are available for both males and females. If you wish, you can even order one that has a brassiere built into it. For more information about these unique undergarments—the cost of which is usually covered by medical insurance—you can write to the Orthotic Undergarment Company and/or Brace Mates. (See Appendix C: Resources.)

One note of caution: Never apply body lotions or petroleum jelly to any part of your skin that is covered by the brace, even if you develop slight sores at points on your body where bones—your hipbones, for example—protrude. Lotions and the like are designed to keep the skin moist and soft, and they will make you more susceptible to sores caused by rubbing. If you must, use rubbing alcohol to soothe these roughened areas. And if the problem persists, make sure you talk to your doctor about it—it may be that your brace doesn't fit properly.

What to Wear Over the Brace

If you are lucky enough to be able to wear an underarm brace, clothing doesn't present much of a problem. Because your neck, shoulders, and chest are free, you can wear the same types of tops you have always worn. But since the pelvic girdle will add about an inch to your waist and hips, be prepared to set aside those skin-tight jeans for a while—you will need slacks that are perhaps one size larger than you're used to. Some young-sters like to wear pants that are elasticized at the waist; they're easier to put on and tend to fit smoothly over the hips. Others who buy fly-front jeans that fit their "new" bodies at the waist and hips often like to have the leg portion taken in so that the pants are properly proportioned all the way down the thighs and legs. You may also want to consider purchasing un-derpants that are large enough to fit *over* your brace. You'll have an easier time removing them when you go to the bathroom.

If you're wearing a Milwaukee brace, you may be worried about how to cover up the neck ring and how to conceal the metal bars in front and back. If you're self-conscious about this, you may want to wear turtleneck tops, or blouses and shirts that are loose-fitting. If wearing such clothing makes you feel better, then go ahead. But bear in mind that a lot of people, sooner or later, don't really care whether they hide the hardware or not. They come to accept that they have to wear the brace, and they just wear clothing that makes them feel comfortable. "I wore turtlenecks all year long," said one young person, "even in hot, muggy weather, in the hope that nobody would find out my secret. But guess what? Most of my friends and acquaintances knew I was wearing a brace, and frankly, they didn't care if they saw a little metal encircling my neck. And after sweating it out for several months, I finally decided that my undercover act just wasn't worth the bother. I wore anything I felt like wearing, including V-neck T-shirts and bare-midriff tops! This 'flaunting' of my brace made me feel better about myself—I was proud that I could endure wearing this con-traption. I was showing the world that I could handle it. And that's some-thing that not everyone can do!"

Maintaining Proper Fit

Once you are wearing your brace, you will be asked to return to the clinic every three or four months so that your doctor can x-ray your spine to see whether or not your curve is progressing, and to see that your brace still fits properly. Since your body will be growing while you are in the brace, it will be necessary for your doctor to adjust the pressure pads and/or the pelvic girdle to accommodate this growth. And if you are wearing a Milwaukee brace, he or she will have to make adjustments to the bars so that they continue to fit as you grow taller. You may even outgrow your brace. If you do, you will have to return to the orthotist for a new one.

Everyday Activities While Wearing the Brace

Many people think that because they are going to be wearing a brace many hours a day for several years, all activity will come to a halt. Nothing could be further from the truth! In fact, exercise is extremely important while you're wearing a brace because it helps to maintain muscle tone.

You will probably meet with a physical therapist after you get your brace. He or she will evaluate your posture, muscles, strength, and flexibility, and talk with you about how active you are right now. Then the therapist will prescribe specific exercises for you to do every day. These may include push-ups while wearing in the brace or pelvic tilts while out of the brace. To do these, you lie on the floor and push the small of your back onto it by tightening your abdominal muscles.

Most doctors encourage people wearing braces to stay active in sports because they are good for your body and great for your psyche as well. Although you should check with your doctor about which sports will be best for you, the following are usually considered acceptable, as long as you don't overexert yourself: tennis, Ping-Pong, running, biking, softball, basketball, volleyball, soccer, golf, rowing, and dancing. With your doctor's permission, you probably will be able to swim (without the brace, of course) each day. It is best to avoid contact sports such as football, hockey, and wrestling—these activities could cause you to hurt yourself or someone else, and you could also damage your brace, which would be costly. If you are skilled at sports such as snow skiing or roller-skating, your doctor may permit you to continue these activities while in your brace.

Weaning from the Brace

From the first day you put on the brace, you will no doubt keep asking your doctor this question: "When can I take it off . . . forever?" His or her answer will depend on your bone age, how long you have worn the brace, whether you've worn it full-time or part-time, and whether or not your curve has progressed during your "confinement."

Let's say that you've been in the brace twenty-three hours a day, every day, for two years, and that by looking at your x-rays your doctor determines that your curve has either stabilized or progressed only slightly. You are now sixteen years old and, from your doctor's predictions, your bones should stop growing within the next year. To see whether you are ready for "weaning," your doctor will take an x-ray of your spine after you have been out of your brace for about two hours. If within those two hours your spine stays in the same position (which your doctor will know because he or she will take another set of x-rays), your doctor will start weaning you from the brace. You will probably be instructed to wear it for twenty-one hours a day for the next three months or so. Then, the next time you come into the office, your doctor will take another x-ray after you have been out of the brace for four hours. If your spine stays the same after this period, your doctor will let you reduce your daily time in the brace to twenty hours. He or she will continue this monitoring every three months, increasing your freedom to twelve and then sixteen hours. At the end of a year, if your spine is still straight after being out of the brace for many hours, you will have to wear it only at night for the last nine months or so. And at the end of that period you'll be free of the brace forever—and chances are good you will have stopped your scoliosis!

Who Pays for the Brace?

If you are lucky, your medical insurance will reimburse you for the price of your brace. In interviewing patients and their parents about braces, however, I learned that insurance companies are becoming increasingly reluctant to cover the cost, or even a portion of the cost, of braces for individuals with adolescent idiopathic scoliosis. This can cause financial difficulty for many, since the price of braces can run from $1,400 to $2,000. Thanks to the members of the Scoliosis Research Society (SRS), however, there is something you can do about this. Charles T. Price, M.D., an orthopedic surgeon at Nemours Children's Clinic in Orlando, Florida, recommends that if your insurance company balks at paying for a brace, you might try forwarding a copy of the recent SRS Position Statement on insurance reimbursement for spinal orthoses (a technical term for appliances worn to straighten the spine, among other things). It makes a strong case for the effectiveness, and the ultimate cost-effectiveness of bracing. (See the boxed inset on page 68.)

What Do Kids Really Think About Braces?

Despite the aggravation that a brace can cause—physically as well as mentally—most youngsters ultimately feel that wearing it was worthwhile, and not just because the brace kept their curves from progressing. In many cases, kids feel that the brace makes them feel stronger psychologically. Take Jan R. for instance. She wore a brace for nearly two years, but it didn't stop her from being nominated for the Junior Horsewoman of the Year Award sponsored by the Horse Show Association in the state where she lives. Says Jan of her experience in the brace, "I think wearing the brace has just made me more determined to succeed at what I do. Wearing it has really taught me a lot about people. I have learned to respect the problems of those who are handicapped and have to spend their lives on crutches or in wheelchairs."

Jan also learned that people can make wearing the brace difficult, but only if you let them. "Don't let it get you down," she says. "People are always ready to feel sorry for you and to baby you, but they don't really know how to let you be yourself and do the things you have to do. The girls in my gymnastics class were amazed that I could touch my toes with my back completely straight." And how did Jan convince her friends that the brace didn't really make her "different"? She says, "You just have to show them that you're still the same person inside you always were."

"No Big Deal"

Seventeen-year-old Vicki J. is the kind of youngster who doesn't let anything—including scoliosis—get her down. In fact, when she met her orthopedist and he told her that she had an S curve, 20 degrees at the top and bottom, she wasn't worried a bit. "The news that I had scoliosis didn't have much of an effect on me," she says. "My curve wasn't very big at first, and my doctor said he'd watch it over the next three months."

When Vicki returned for x-rays three months later, her curve had indeed increased: the top now measured 29 degrees; the bottom, 21. "The doctor showed me a little model of an underarm brace," she says. "The thought of wearing it didn't bother me at all. It was no big deal.

"It didn't bother me to have to wear the brace to school. Nobody ever made fun of me that I can remember, but the first day I wore it, kids at school seemed scared to say anything to me. Eventually word got around behind my back that I was wearing a brace because I had scoliosis, and then I was treated just like everybody else.

"I have to admit it: sometimes it made me feel self-conscious. But it also gave me an excuse. Sometimes teenagers feel like they have to do everything that everybody else is doing; they feel like they have to be part of the crowd. When I didn't want to be part of the crowd, or if I wasn't

SRS Position Statement:
Insurance Reimbursement for Spinal Orthosis
Used in the Treatment of Idiopathic Scoliosis

Brace treatment for idiopathic scoliosis in growing children is an established nonsurgical method for reducing the risk of scoliosis progression. Based upon current evidence, it is the opinion of the Scoliosis Research Society that bracing reduces the incidence of surgery for scoliosis.

Studies of bracing efficacy have demonstrated that patients who do not wear braces are three to four times more likely to require spinal fusion surgery than similar groups of braced patients. Third-party payers should note that bracing for scoliosis is used for prevention of progressive, disabling deformity. Bracing is frequently a medically necessary component of the treatment of scoliosis. Spinal orthoses for scoliosis should not be considered "durable medical equipment" similar to wheelchairs, handrails, hospital beds, and other items that may assist in the performance of normal activities of daily living. Third-party payers should recognize that bracing for scoliosis is cost-effective since it can reduce the need for expensive surgical intervention.

Furthermore, multiple spinal orthoses may be required during the period of growth when scoliosis requires treatment. Restrictions on the number of braces in a year or over several years may have a detrimental effect on the end result of nonoperative management for idiopathic scoliosis.

It is in the best interests of the patients and also cost-effective for the third party payers to provide reimbursement for spinal orthoses when prescribed by the treating physician for the complete management of idiopathic scoliosis.

REFERENCES

N.J. Allington and J.R. Bowen, "Adolescent Idiopathic Scoliosis: Treatment with the Wilmington Brace. A Comparison of Full-Time and Part-Time Use," *Journal of Bone and Joint Surgery* (American Volume) 78 (7) (July 1996): 1056–1062.

J.B. Emans, A. Kaelin, P. Bancel, J.E. Hall, and M.E. Miller, "The Boston Bracing System for Idiopathic Scoliosis. Follow-up Results in 295 Patients," *Spine* 11 (8) (October 1986): 792–801.

R. Fernandez-Feliberti, J. Flynn, N. Ramirez, M. Trautmann, and M. Alegria, "Effectiveness of TLSO bracing in the Conservative Treatment of Idiopathic Scoliosis," *Journal of Pediatric Orthopedics* 15 (2) (March–April 1995): 176–181.

A.L. Nachemson and L.E. Peterson, "Effectiveness of Treatment with a Brace in Girls Who Have Adolescent Idiopathic Scoliosis. A prospective, controlled study based on data from the Brace Study of the Scoliosis Research Society," *Journal of Bone and Joint Surgery* 77 (6) (June 1995): 815–822.

C.T. Price, D.S. Scott, F.R. Reed, J.T. Sproul, and M.F. Riddick, "Nighttime Bracing for Adolescent Idiopathic Scoliosis with the Charleston Bending Brace: Long-Term Follow-up," *Journal of Pediatric Orthopedics* 17 (6) (November–December 1997): 703–707.

D.E. Rowe, S.M. Bernstein, M.F. Riddick, F. Adler, J.B. Emans, and D. Gardner-Bonneau, "A Meta-Analysis of the Efficacy of Non-Operative Treatments for Idiopathic Scoliosis," *Journal of Bone and Joint Surgery* 79 (5) (May 1997): 664–674.

feeling too popular anyway, I could always blame the brace. I know it was unrealistic to think that way, but somehow it helped me feel better about myself when I was feeling insecure or unpopular.

"I didn't give up any activities because of the brace. I took dancing—ballet, tap, and jazz. I got permission from my orthopedist to take off the brace for an hour during the day so I could practice dancing. He said the exercise would help strengthen my back. I even started cheerleading while I was in it. I didn't do anything incredibly daring, mind you, but I could do most of the cheers and some of the jumps. Of course, sometimes the brace got in my way—like the first time I tried to play softball in it. The coach put me out in center field and the batter hit a grounder to me. I squatted down and fell face first in the dirt! It was the most embarrassing moment of my life! But I'd probably have felt that way even if I hadn't been wearing a brace at the time.

"In the three years and two months that I wore the brace, the only thing that bugged me was how my parents and grandparents would sometimes treat me. They'd give me special treatment. If I bent over to pick something up, they say, 'Oh, don't do that, you'll hurt your back.' I guess they thought I wasn't capable of doing normal things. But I just felt like I could do anything! And I pretty much did everything I wanted to. I just had to show them that I wasn't an invalid.

"Today my curves are 21 and 17, and I don't have to wear the brace anymore. I feel good and look good. The brace made me feel better about myself, because it's not something everybody can get through."

A Love-Hate Relationship

Although she's now in her thirties, Marsha P. has no trouble recalling what it was like wearing her Milwaukee brace from 1977 to 1980, when all youngsters wore braces for twenty-three hours per day. Her story begins in 1976, when she was in sixth grade:

"I didn't know anything about scoliosis then. In fact, on the day that the school nurse screened us, I didn't have any idea why I was being asked to bend over. She checked out my back and then called in another nurse. They mumbled something about my having a slight curvature, but said it was probably nothing to worry about. I took their word for it.

"By the time I was in seventh grade I knew a little bit about scoliosis. One of the girls in my class was wearing a back brace, and we all knew it was because she had a curvature in her spine. So when it came time to be screened that year, I had some idea of what they were looking for when they asked me to bend over. Of course, I was afraid that if they found a curvature, I'd have to wear a brace just like hers.

"When the exam was over, the nurse told me she thought I had scoliosis, and that she'd be sending a letter home to my mother. I came home bawling that day—I thought for sure I had it. I felt terrible!

"But when we got the letter, all it said was that in scoliosis screening they noticed I had something called a *thoracic hump*. That was all the letter said. I thought to myself, 'Oh, this is something different. This isn't scoliosis.' I tried to talk myself out of it, I guess, and I told kids at school that it wasn't scoliosis after all. But when we went to my family doctor, he took an x-ray. Sure enough, I had scoliosis. I was devastated. All I could think about was I'd have to wear a brace. So my mom and I made an appointment with a specialist to find out what would have to happen next.

"I was pretty nervous when I met the specialist, but he tried to reassure me by saying that just because I had scoliosis, it didn't mean I'd have to wear a brace. He said he'd take an x-ray of my spine to see how it looked. Then all of us together would decide what to do.

"When the x-ray came back from the lab, the doctor put it up to the light and I could see the curve for myself. I was really upset, because I felt fine, yet I could see how my spine had curved into an S shape. I couldn't feel it, but there it was, crooked! He explained that because both parts of the curve measured 26 degrees—the top and bottom—it was a 'balanced' curve. He said it wasn't that bad, and that we wouldn't have to do anything for now. We could come back in three months, and he'd check it again to see if it had gotten worse. I was so relieved! Maybe I wouldn't have to wear a brace after all!

"When we went back to his office three months later, I had more x-rays taken. My curve had gotten bigger—the top was now 36 degrees, and the bottom was 18 degrees. Now my curve was unbalanced. And because it had increased in just three months, it would probably keep getting worse—unless I was put into a Milwaukee brace.

"As soon as he said that, I wanted to bawl my head off. I was really scared! I didn't want to have any part of it at all. I figured that if I had to wear it, nobody would like me. As a seventh grader, I was just starting to realize that boys were pretty interesting, and I figured if I had to wear a brace, I'd never have a boyfriend. That seems silly to me now, but then it was really important.

"I kept thinking about that girl who wore a brace at school. Everybody thought she was weird—mostly because she had a terrible personality—but I really thought people would think of me the same way. I didn't get much time to dwell on that, because before I knew it, I was being fitted for the brace.

"They had a lot of trouble fitting the brace to me. I spent an entire day going between the doctor and the brace people, what with all the adjustments they had to make. Then they gave me the wrong brace—it belonged to another girl, but nobody knew it for several hours. They kept trying to adjust it to fit me, but of course it wouldn't. Finally somebody figured out that they had the wrong brace, and they finally located the one that was intended for me. By the time they all finished working me over, I was really uncomfortable, but at least it fit!

"I felt so awkward trying to get into the car to go home. I couldn't just hop in the way I used to. Now I had to sort of slide into the seat, and when I finally got in, I felt like I couldn't breathe—that neck ring really pinched me under the chin! All the way home I stared at the ceiling of the car and wondered how I'd ever get used to wearing this thing. How would I ever face the kids at school?

"When I woke up the next morning, I took one look at the brace and decided no way, I just could not face the idea of having to go to school with it. It was almost the end of the school year, and I thought if I could just avoid wearing it for another month or so, nobody would ever have to know.

"Mom and I fought constantly. At first she tried being sympathetic about it. She'd say, 'I know you don't like this. I understand, but you've just got to wear it.' I refused to listen to her. I simply wasn't going to wear it.

"Finally, just to keep the peace, I agreed to wear it—but only when I slept. Mom got so frustrated with me that she called the clinic and got the names of twin girls who'd had scoliosis and worn braces, and she made me go over to their house to talk. I think she thought this would make me feel better—seeing other girls who had the same problem—but actually it didn't help me much. As it turned out, the girls had just gotten out of their braces. There they sat, with perfectly straight backs and no braces. That would never be me, I thought. And besides, they were seventeen. I was twelve. I had such a long time to go!

"After that, my mom tried again to help. This time she found a young woman in her twenties who'd had surgery for scoliosis and arranged for us to have dinner together. Maybe she thought it would scare me into wearing the brace.

"That was the first time I'd worn the brace out in public. Talking to that woman didn't really help me, but getting out did. I kept thinking everybody in the restaurant was staring at me, but after a while it didn't bother me as much. That was the best thing I could have done—making the first move to wear it outside and seeing people's reaction to it. That summer I occasionally wore the brace in public, but I still wore it mostly when I slept.

"When I started eighth grade that fall, I had resolved that I was going to have to wear it because it wasn't going to go away. That first day of eighth grade was the hardest of my life, because I knew if I didn't wear it that day, I never would.

"I got through the first day all right, and then everything was okay. I wore turtlenecks to try and hide it as much as possible, but the kids at school could still see it underneath my clothes. They weren't negative about it at all—just inquisitive. Everybody wanted to know what it was for, and how I could sleep with it on. As time went on, more and more people knew about it, and I eventually quit trying to hide it with clothes. I became bolder and just didn't care about it that much.

"I wore the brace pretty regularly during eighth and ninth grade, and finally, when I started tenth grade, the doctor said I could be weaned from it. My curves were now at 25 and 18 degrees, and they stabilized even when I was out of the brace for hours at a time. For several months I only had to wear it for sixteen hours a day. Eventually I only had to wear it at night.

"At last the day came when my orthopedist said I didn't have to wear it anymore. You'd think I would have been ecstatic about it, but I wasn't! I'd gotten so used to sleeping with it on that I couldn't bear to be without it! Would you believe I still continued wearing it at night for three more whole months? I'd really gotten to like the support the brace gave me. In fact, I felt like I was melting into the bed without it. I actually couldn't fall asleep without it!

"When I told my doctor about it, he put his foot down and said I couldn't be so dependent on the brace, that eventually I'd get used to sleeping without it. Of course he was right, but I sure had a hard time going along with it. When I visited the clinic, I came to be known as the girl who liked her brace so much she didn't want to take it off.

"It seems funny now, especially since I had so much trouble getting used to the brace in the beginning. But I think the whole experience taught me a lot about myself. Wearing a brace made me go through something at a young age—it was something I *had* to accept. A lot of kids aren't faced with something hard like that. But I was forced to deal with it and had to learn to look at the good side of things. I couldn't just sit there and feel sorry for myself. I finally had to realize that it was still me inside the brace, that it didn't really matter. It helped to talk to people about it, to explain things to them. Once you bring it out in the open, it makes it easier for you and for them."

TEARS FIRST, THEN ACCEPTANCE

Diane B. has had more than her share of medical problems. When she was only a year and a half old, she had surgery to repair a hip that was dislocated at birth. Later, she developed kidney infections that would plague her for several of her childhood years. When she was screened for scoliosis in sixth grade, at age twelve, the school nurse noticed that one of her shoulders seemed higher than the other. "It looked like I had a lump on my back," recalls Diane, "and I immediately thought it was cancer. I'd had so many problems with my body up to that point, it wouldn't have surprised me if it had been cancer. Even so, I was really scared!"

Diane and her parents made an appointment with the family doctor, who assured them that Diane's problem wasn't cancer. It was scoliosis. He referred them to a scoliosis specialist in another city. Diane had x-rays taken; then came the verdict: She had a 21-degree curvature. "It was just another blow," says Diane's mother, Pat. "Diane had had so many medical problems, all of them major. But each problem had been corrected, and we just hoped that this one would follow the same path."

When the orthopedist told the family that Diane would have to wear a brace for several years to keep the curve from progressing, Diane burst into tears. "It was really difficult for me to accept. Since I'd had this history of problems, it seemed like everything about me was bad. This was just one more problem, and I kept wondering, 'Why me?' I kept right on crying as my parents tried to comfort me. They kept trying to make me feel better by reminding me that some kids can't walk, some kids have braces on their teeth. And they tried to encourage me by saying that if the doctor could help me in some way, I should take him up on it. I knew they were right, but I didn't like hearing about it. Why did I have to go through this?

"I was pretty self-conscious wearing the brace during the first week of school, but my friends and teachers pretty much accepted it. Since everybody in school knew about the brace anyway, I eventually quit trying to hide it. Another girl in my class wore one, but she'd always try to cover hers and pretend it wasn't there. She wouldn't talk to people about it. I could see she was making things uncomfortable for herself and other people, and I didn't want that to happen to me. So I was pretty open about it, and that helped a lot.

"I kept active while I was wearing the brace. I'd play softball with it on and even wore it on a trip to Hawaii. In fact, I got to the point where I felt best with it on—I'd feel like a noodle when I took it off.

"Each time I returned to the clinic, the curve had gotten progressively worse. When it reached 40 degrees—what all the doctors call the 'magic number'—I started to worry that I might have to have surgery. That was a big fear, so I did my brace exercises a ton of times, hoping they'd help. I think they did, because my curve has stayed right around 40 degrees to this day.

"My parents really helped me through it. They always went with me to the doctor and would encourage me to do my exercises and to wear the brace twenty-three hours a day. They kept telling me the doctor knew what he was doing, and that the brace would help me. If they would have questioned it, I would have, too. But they accepted it, and so did I.

"A lot of my parents' friends would say to them, 'How can you make your daughter wear it?' But Mom and Dad would say, 'You don't know Diane. She's got a great attitude and she can handle it.' It made me feel good to know they had a lot of confidence in me. I might have had some real serious psychological problems if it hadn't been for them."

These are some typical reactions of young people who have had to wear braces to combat scoliosis. It can be uncomfortable, especially at first, but bracing is an effective treatment for many people with idiopathic scoliosis. However, if curvature exceeds 40 degrees, surgery is likely to be recommended. In the following chapter, we will look at surgical options for treating and correcting scoliosis.

Surgical Treatments

For Adolescents and Adults with Curves
of 40 Degrees and Beyond

This chapter examines the surgical techniques that are available today. It will provide you with a fairly graphic picture of what orthopedic surgeons actually do in the operating room in the process of straightening out spinal curves. In Chapter 5, you will meet youngsters and adults who have had operations to correct their scoliosis, and they will tell you about their surgical experience in their own words. In most cases, they are extremely candid about their emotions, frustrations, and pain, both psychological and physical.

Before you delve into this chapter, however, you need to know that your state of mind can have an important effect on the amount of distress you experience before and after surgery, and that it can even affect your rate of recovery. Some people find that knowing all there is to know about surgery improves their state of mind. It makes them feel that they're in control of the situation. For others, the motto "Ignorance is bliss" holds true—the less they know about the surgery, the better they can cope with it. If you belong in the second category, skip this chapter and move on to the next.

A Historical Perspective

Before we explore the most common procedures used today, let's step back in time—to 1911, when Russell Hibbs, an orthopedic surgeon at the New York Orthopaedic Hospital in New York City, performed the world's first spinal fusion. To find out about the early days of spine surgery, I asked Dr. Hugo Keim—now retired from that hospital—to provide a bit of history.

It seems unbelievable that anyone even considered doing spine surgery in 1911. Doctors then just used "drop" ether, and that didn't always keep the patient asleep. They had no blood-replacement products and no antibiotics to guard against infection. In fact, when Dr. Hibbs proposed the idea of doing a spine fusion on a person who had tuberculosis, everybody thought he was a maniac. He wasn't allowed to become a member of the American Orthopaedic Association—the members blackballed him because they thought he was crazy!

Hibbs didn't use rods and wire fixations—he just fused the spine. But because he had no way to keep the spine straight while it healed— the job that rods and wires do today—he took two or three vertebrae at a time, welding them together by using little chips of bone taken from the spine. This meant that he had to bring a patient into surgery, do two or three fusions, close up the incisions, put her in a plaster cast, and keep her in the hospital for six to eight weeks while she healed. Then he'd have to go back in and do another two or three vertebrae, finish the job, put on another cast, leave her on her back for another six to eight weeks, and repeat this routine until all of the curved vertebrae were fused. Believe it or not, the average patient in those days was here in the hospital for a whole year!

Russell Hibbs paved the way for the kinds of spine operations we do today. Although he was initially considered a complete wacko by his peers, his pioneering work as a surgeon would eventually be hailed as brilliant, and the medical community realized that much could be learned from him.

Surgeons today owe a great debt to Dr. Hibbs, but as you will see, they have added some highly sophisticated techniques to spinal fusions. As a result, spine surgery today is far more complex—and more successful—than at any other time in history.

The Evolution of Internal Fixation

In order to hold the spine in place while the fusion heals to form a straighter spine, surgeons use a technique called internal fixation, which involves the implantation of metal instrumentation around the spinal column. Spinal instrumentation may consist of hooks, rods, screws, and/or wires, depending on an individual's particular requirements. The hardware allows the surgeon to reduce and/or adjust the curvature to some degree. To keep the curve from progressing, the surgeon then performs a spinal fusion and may utilize bone grafts from the iliac crest of the hipbone, or may use bone from a bone bank or collagraft bone substitutes. Eventually, the grafted bone fuses into a solid bone mass, and the vertebrae are permanently immobilized—a process that can take up to a year or more in adults. During this healing period, instrumentation is used to make the spine stiff and hold it so that the fusion can set. Once the fusion solidifies, the hardware is no longer needed and can be removed, although usually it is left in place. If the fusion is not solid—a condition known as *pseudoarthrosis*—the hardware will eventually become fatigued and fail.

To better understand modern instrumentation, it's helpful to take a quick look at how it has evolved since the 1940s, when Dr. Paul Harrington of Houston, Texas, developed the Harrington rod system. Although he was not the first to propose the use of metal fixation, his spinal hardware represents the first generation of instrumentation and has been used for decades.

First Generation:
The Harrington Rod Technique

The Harrington rod system employed a thin metal rod inserted on the concave side of the curve and corrected the curve through "distraction"—a way of pulling the ends of the curve farther apart. (See Figure 4.1.) Using a number of hooks, plus a device that operated much like a car jack, a surgeon would ratchet the spine to a point at which he was satisfied with the correction. Patients with Harrington rods usually wore braces for six months or more after the operation.

Although it was considered the safest technique at the time, the major drawback of the Harrington rod system was that it allowed little restoration of the normal contours of the spine when viewed from the side, in-

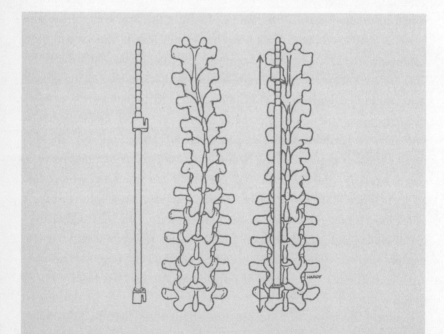

Figure 4.1. The Harrington rod implant was the first generation of spinal instrumentation for idiopathic scoliosis. The Harrington distraction rod lengthens the curve.

cluding the normal outward curve at the top of the spine—kyphosis—and the normal inward curve at the bottom—lordosis—both of which are typically distorted by scoliosis. Today, a problem known as *flat-back syndrome* (see page 96) is often blamed on the use of distraction with the Harrington technique. The Harrington rod system also was not as stable as modern devices are, so there was a higher incidence of pseudoarthrosis.

SECOND GENERATION:
THE DWYER, ZIELKE, AND LUQUE TECHNIQUES

In the 1960s, Australian orthopedic surgeon Alan Dwyer and Dr. Klaus Zielke of Germany each pioneered the anterior approach to surgery, which involved removing some of the intervertebral discs to make a curve more flexible and easier to correct. With the Dwyer technique, instead of distracting the spine and fusing all the vertebrae involved in the curve, the surgeon removed several discs located between vertebrae at the top, or apex, of a curve, inserted bone graft into the remaining spaces, and compressed the outer edges of these vertebrae with a special cable system that derotated and straightened the spine. The Zielke system mimicked the Dwyer, but used a flexible rod instead of a cable and employed a special tool that helped the surgeon derotate the spine while straightening the curve. (See Figure 4.2.) Postoperative braces were generally used. The major drawback of both the Dwyer and Zielke systems was that they corrected only one plane and had a tendency to produce flat-back syndrome.

About a decade later, Dr. Eduardo Luque of Mexico City developed a technique known as *sublaminar wiring*. He used two flexible L-shaped rods placed on either side of the spine. The rods were contoured to conform to the curve, and wires were threaded through the spinal canal at each vertebral level. The wires were then twisted around the rods on either side of the spine, applying pressure on the spine to correct the curve. (See Figure 4.3.) Because there are multiple points of fixation, patients generally did not have to wear a postoperative brace. The major drawback with the Luque system was that, since the wires passed through the spinal

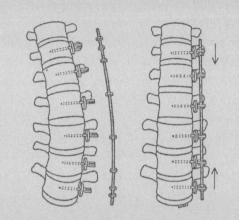

Figure 4.2. When a Zielke implant is used, a flexible rod is threaded through the tops of screws inserted into the vertebrae. A special attachment (not shown) derotates and straightens the spine.

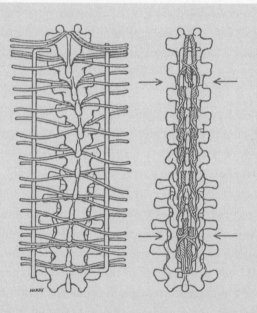

Figure 4.3. A Luque-type implant consists of two L-shaped rods, plus many wires that are passed through the neural or spinal canal. When wiring is complete, the ends are twisted and turned down.

canal, there was a greater risk of neurological damage than with other systems. Some surgeons today still use a Luque-type system to treat patients whose bones are very fragile, which makes attachment of hardware through hooks or screws difficult.

THIRD GENERATION: THE COTREL-DUBOUSSET SYSTEM

In 1984, Dr. Yves Cotrel and Dr. Jean Dubousset of France introduced the Cotrel-Dubousset (C-D) instrumentation, a system that employed the best part of the Harrington—its safety factor—with the best of the Luque—the strength from two rods and an increased number of attachment points. The original C-D was hailed as an extremely stable implant technique that not only corrected a curve from the front and side, but also derotated it. However, the first C-D devices had a tendency to produce an imbalance by overcorrecting one curve and therefore producing more deformity. Today, variations on the original C-D are able to deal with types of scoliosis that were not addressed by earlier internal fixation techniques.

Spinal Instrumention for the New Millennium

Surgeons today use a variety of what are called *multiple segmental instrumentation techniques* to treat scoliotic curves. Some surgeons use their own modern variations on the C-D; others employ the Texas Scottish Rite Hospital (TSRH) system. Some prefer the Isola system, designed by Dr. Marc Asher and Dr. Charles Heinig and engineers Walter Strippgen and Dr. William Carson. Other techniques—among them the Moss Miami and Paragon—are available as well.

Why is multiple segmental instrumentation so popular? First, let's go to the spine for an answer. When the spine curves sideways, the vertebrae rotate toward the concavity (inside) of the curve. Because the ribs are attached to the spine, they are pulled along and become splayed out on the convex (outward) side of the curve while being compressed on the concave side—a situation that creates the rib hump seen in some people with thoracic curves.

The newer instrumentation systems, which can be modified for use in either posterior or anterior procedures, allow the surgeon to bend or contour the rods to conform to the desired profile. The rods are positioned on either side of the spine and affixed to the vertebrae with multiple hooks and sometimes screws as well. The rods themselves are joined to each other by transverse rods or connecting devices.

According to Dr. David Bradford, the most important facet of the TSRH, Isola, and others is the fact that they have the ability to control not just the compression or distraction, and not just to correct scoliosis, but also to build in correction of lordosis and kyphosis. Further, he notes: "The newer devices have a better construct and you can correct the spine in two or three planes. We're getting superb correction and can maintain it and also prevent secondary deformities from occurring. The systems are lower profile than ever before, and far less bulky."

How do the systems differ? Primarily in the ways in which the hooks are attached to the rods. The C-D, for example, uses a setscrew; the TSRH is a nut-and-bolt arrangement; and the Isola utilizes a drop set-in screw. Basically, however, they all work on the same principle and accomplish the same ends. Because they provide a very stable fixation, they usually do not require a postoperative brace—but, as always, you should let your doctor be your guide.

The Spinal Fusion

The major component of most scoliosis operations is the spinal fusion—the transformation of a movable portion of the spine into a solid mass of bone. How do surgeons perform this feat?

After the instrumentation is in place, the surgeon prepares the spine for the bone graft that will fuse to it by removing the outer bone, or *cortex,* of each vertebra involved in the curve. By decorticating the vertebrae, the surgeon can expose the living bone underneath. This is a spongy, porous sort of bone that releases blood, the life-giving ingredient that will help your spine—and the bone graft that is going to be inserted—fuse together into a solid piece of bone.

Bone graft can be gotten in two ways. With a special tool, a surgeon can harvest small strips of bone from the hip or ribs. The bone is then cut into hundreds of matchstick-sized strips, which are packed in a crisscross fashion from the top to the bottom of the decorticated vertebrae. In many cases, the surgeon may instead opt to use bone from a bone bank, referred to as *allograft*. But that's not all. According to Dr. Frank Rand, an orthopedic surgeon at New England Baptist Hospital in Boston, there are now genetically engineered bone proteins that may also be added to the mix. Known as *osteoinductive compounds* and *bone morphogenic proteins*, these can stimulate the body to produce a stronger fusion.

After four to six months, for adolescents, and six to twelve months or longer, for adults, the fusion melds together into one solid piece of bone. Says Dr. Hugo Keim of the eventual fusion: "It's beautiful. It looks like someone poured molten wax over the spine. You cannot distinguish between the individual strips of bone. What you really end up with is a single, smooth, elongated section of vertebrae."

In the future, says Dr. Rand, the process of fusing the spine will become even more sophisticated: "During surgery, we'll be able to put in a harmless local infection with a benign adenovirus [a common type of virus] that that will crank out bone morphogenic proteins for months and weeks and induce a fusion. The use of blood platelet-derived growth factors is on the horizon, too; we'll sprinkle them along the fused area to enhance healing."

Deciding to Have Surgery

If your doctor has recommended surgery for your scoliosis, he or she will do a spinal fusion with instrumentation that aims to accomplish four goals:

1. To correct your deformity;
2. To straighten and stabilize the spine;
3. To prevent further progression and/or deterioration; and
4. To alleviate pain or discomfort.

Of course, the ultimate decision as to whether to have surgery is up to you. But to make the best choice possible, it is important to talk with your doctor, ask questions, and, if you wish, to obtain a second opinion. As you gather information, take your time—scoliosis surgery is not emergency surgery—and finally ask yourself: What is likely to happen if I do have surgery, and what is likely to happen if I don't? Weigh the pros against the cons, make an inventory of how surgery may or may not change your quality of life (physically, emotionally, and psychologically), and discuss any and all concerns with your doctor and parents or other loved ones. Eventually, you will come to a decision that's right for you.

If you decide to go through with surgery, you will begin to hear your doctor talk about the two approaches to scoliosis surgery available today: posterior (referring to the back of the spine) and anterior (meaning the front of the spine). With the posterior approach, surgeons make an incision down the middle of the back; with the anterior, they make an incision along the right or left side of the body, depending upon the direction of the curve. To help explain why a surgeon today may choose to do one approach or another—or both—I interviewed Dr. Howard King, an orthopedic spine surgeon at Inter-Mountain Orthopedics in Boise, Idaho, who shared answers to the kinds of questions most of his patients ask.

Q: *Is the surgical procedure the same for the posterior and anterior approaches?*

A: Scoliosis surgery involves straightening the curve and stabilizing the spine, either with bone grafts (fusion) or spine instrumentation, and in most cases, both. These steps are essentially the same for posterior and anterior surgery. The primary difference is that in the anterior approach, we have access to the larger part of the vertebra for fixation of spine instrumentation, and we can also remove the discs in between the vertebrae to free up the spine and gain better correction.

Q: *Can anterior surgery be used in all situations?*

A: No, it's not indicated in all situations. Additionally, it is a more complex procedure and therefore has more potential risk. In scoliosis surgery, our goal is to get the best correction and stability we can while fusing the fewest vertebral segments possible and minimizing surgical and postsurgical complications. Using different approaches or a combination of them helps us to achieve that goal.

Q: *Generally speaking, when do surgeons use the posterior approach and when do they opt for anterior?*

A: For scoliosis, posterior surgery is primarily for single thoracic and double (thoracic/lumbar) curves. Anterior surgery may be used for a lumbar or thoraco-lumbar curve. Recently, anterior instrumentation and fusion have been done for thoracic curves.

Q: *Under what circumstances would you do both anterior and posterior procedures?*

A: We would do both procedures on someone who has a very large, stiff, rigid curve—a situation in which we are trying to help the person gain spine correction. We'd also do both on an adult who needed a very long fusion down to the pelvis, and on a young child who has a lot of growth left. We would also do both procedures on someone with significant kyphosis [see page 14]; the combination of the two approaches would give the best correction and stability.

Q: *Why would anterior/posterior surgery be done on a young, growing child?*

A: In a young, growing child, we want to avoid what's known as "crankshafting." If a child is very young—eight or nine—and has not yet gone through his or her rapid-growth phase, posterior fusion alone would stop the growth of the posterior portion of the spine, but the anterior portion would continue to grow and the scoliosis would continue to worsen. The anterior technique would be done to arrest that anterior growth.

Q: *When you do both procedures, do you do them in stages a few days apart, or on the same day?*

A: If we were faced with a really complicated reconstruction, we might opt to do it in stages. But generally speaking, we usually do both procedures on the same day. We start with the anterior portion to free up to the spine, and then continue with the posterior portion.

Q: *What is the advantage of doing both procedures on the same day?*

A: One advantage is it reduces the overall time that the patient is under anesthesia, and that helps to reduce recovery time. By doing both procedures on the same day, we can also reduce the amount of time the patient spends in the hospital. With surgeries on the same day, a patient might spend five days in the hospital, versus two weeks for a patient who has the surgeries in stages. We also know from good studies that postoperative nutrition and blood-clotting factors are better with same day procedures.

Q: *Do you decide on the approach(es) on a case-by-case basis?*

A: Absolutely. When it comes to surgery for scoliosis, every case is different—no one particular approach will work for everyone.

Although many surgeons perform posterior fusions on people with congenital scoliosis, Dr. Ronald Moskovich, an orthopedic surgeon affiliated with the Hospital for Joint Diseases in New York City, is one of a handful of doctors who are taking a more aggressive approach—operating on both the front *and* back of the spine and removing the problematic vertebrae. "The kids tolerate it very well," he notes, "and we get a fairly normal pattern of growth without the risk of the child developing further scoliosis later in life."

A New Approach: Endoscopic Surgery

Surgical patients have always hoped that surgeons would develop a minimally invasive approach to scoliosis surgery—a technique that would result in a smaller incision and a less obvious scar while effectively and safely correcting a curvature. Thanks to the pioneering work of orthopedic spine surgeons including Dr. Ronald Blackman, Head of Spine Service at Children's Hospital in Oakland, California; Dr. George Picetti of Kaiser Permanente medical center; and Dr. Eduardo Luque of Mexico, the endoscopic technique for scoliosis surgery is doing just that.

The endoscope is an instrument that has a small video camera attached to it. When inserted into a cavity such as the chest (after the lung has been carefully collapsed), the endoscope allows the surgeon to see the contents of this cavity, which includes the front part of the spine—the vertebral bodies—on a video screen. Then, using specially made instruments that are inserted through small portholes roughly one inch in length, the surgeon operates while viewing his or her movements on the screen. Since the mid-1990s, some surgeons have used the endoscopic technique to make small incisions into the side of the chest to remove discs to loosen up the spine prior to doing a posterior fusion. But with the new work being done by Dr. Blackman and others, he notes that the endoscope can be used to visualize placing screws into each of the involved vertebral bodies and connecting the screws to a rod to actually correct the spine through these small incisions.

Today, the technique is used primarily on individuals with curves in the upper or thoracic area, but it is also occasionally used on people with thoracolumbar curves. It works best on adolescents who have curves that are around 45 degrees or less, and quite flexible. The need to deflate and reinflate the lung poses no problems—in fact, heart surgeons have used this procedure for years without mishap.

As to the potential for crankshaft phenomenon as a result of fusing the anterior spine only, Dr. Blackman says that fusing anteriorly should actually *prevent* crankshafting. There does not appear to be a reverse phenomenon in which the back continues to grow when the front is solid, at least in adolescents.

With anterior endoscopic surgery, doctors often fuse two or three fewer vertebrae than they would with standard posterior surgery. This leaves patients with a bit more of a curve, but with greater flexibility in the lumbar spine, which is something most sixteen- to eighteen-year-olds find desirable. As to what may happen to a curve twenty or more years after this treatment, doctors do not yet know. It is possible that a second procedure might be necessary much later, but as Dr. Blackman notes, if we can avoid going into the lumbar spine for the next twenty or so years, that should be better than fusing the vertebrae all the way down.

Endoscopic surgery also requires a shorter recovery period. On average, patients are out of bed one to two days after surgery and leave the hospital within three to four days. They also have less discomfort and come off pain medication sooner.

"It's a promising technique," says Dr. Blackman, "but we need more long-term results to determine if and when this approach will be considered as good or better than standard surgery. Right now, we're encouraged enough to continue using it on certain patients, but we'll continue making changes to improve the technique."

Rib Thoracoplasty Surgery

If you have a rib hump, you may want to talk to a surgeon about having a procedure known as *rib thoracoplasty*. This is a surgical technique that involves the shortening of certain ribs in the thoracic or chest area. The procedure is done to reduce the size and severity of a rib hump that may accompany scoliosis. It is usually performed after corrective surgery for scoliosis.

To find out more about rib thoracoplasty, I consulted with Dr. Serena S. Hu, an orthopedic surgeon at the University of California. What follows are excerpts of the discussion:

Q: *What are the goals of a rib thoracoplasty?*

A: For moderately severe deformities, the procedure appears to result in a significantly greater improvement in a patient's overall appearance though it will not result in perfect symmetry. The procedure also relieves pain that may be associated with a rib hump, such as when an individual leans up against a chair.

Q: *Are there different surgical techniques being used today for rib thoracoplasty?*

A: Most surgeons use fairly similar techniques. However, some surgeons make an incision over the peak of the rib hump, whereas I prefer, as do many others, to use a midline incision— that is, to use the same incision that's used for a posterior spinal fusion. Patients seem to prefer having a single midline incision.

Q: *What determines which ribs are shortened, and how do you decide how much to shorten them?*

A: We determine which ribs are shortened based on which ones are prominent and are not expected to be reduced by correction of the curvature. As far as deciding how much to shorten ribs, we decide on a case-by-case basis. It depends on the nature of a patient's curve, as well as on the severity of the rib hump.

Q: *When the ribs grow back after surgery, do they actually form new rib bone and reconnect to the spine? How long does it take for this to happen?*

A: Yes, the ribs do grow back, forming a new rib. This takes approximately two to three months.

Q: *Is the new growth as strong as the original rib?*

A: Once it is completely healed, the new rib will be a strong as the original rib.

Q: *Is there any chance of the rib hump returning?*

A: That would occur only if the curvature progressed.

Q: *Can a rib grow back crooked or out of place?*
A: This is rarely, if ever, encountered.

Q: *Is it always necessary to wear a brace following this surgery? Will wearing one or not affect the outcome of the surgery?*
A: The use of a brace appears to protect the ribs from rubbing against the chest cavity and seems to result in less likelihood of fluid collection and the subsequent need for a chest tube. Not wearing a brace will not affect the long-term outcome of the surgery, but in the short term, a brace could avoid the complications mentioned.

Q: *During recovery, is there any danger for the unprotected chest wall?*
A: Not in the course of normal activities. There might be a theoretical risk of a very forceful blunt trauma causing damage, but this would, of course, be very unusual.

Q: *Can a patient damage the rib cage during recovery by stretching or moving incorrectly? Are there any movement restrictions once the healing is complete?*
A: A patient wouldn't damage the rib cage during the course of normal activities. Once healing is complete, there are no movement restrictions. In fact, tennis and golf could be possible with the constraints of spine fusion limitations.

Q: *How long is the recovery time?*
A: For patients who choose to undergo thoracoplasty surgery as a separate procedure, the full time in the hospital is five to seven days, and recovery is two to three months for this procedure.

Q: *Aside from the risks of anesthesia, what are the possible complications from this procedure and what can be done about them?*
A: The main complications would be fluid or air collecting in the lungs. Either of these situations can be treated with a device

called a chest tube. There might be too much resection, resulting in a rib concavity, and there could be a temporary decrease
of lung capacity.

Q: *Can a patient go back to surgery after the corrective spine surgery
and have a rib thoracoplasty?*
A: Yes. Many patients elect to have the thoracoplasty performed
after recovery from their major spinal corrective surgery.

Revision Surgery

Sometimes, people who went through scoliosis surgery earlier in life suffer from problems later on. Possible longer-term problems after scoliosis
surgery include pseudoarthrosis (failure of the bone graft to heal), pain
from the hardware, progressive deformities above or below the original fusion, and disc degeneration. To correct such problems, surgeons may do
revision or reconstruction surgery. To find out more about it, I consulted
with Dr. Frank Rand, who specializes in revision surgery.

Q: *When problems occur after a patient's original surgery, what do
you typically do?*
A: Revision surgery may involve repair work on the original fusion,
but more often it involves problems just below the original fusion surgery. Problems that occur within the zone of the original
surgery include repair of a pseudoarthrosis. Problems that occur
just below the original surgery include spinal stenosis [narrow-
ing of the opening(s) through which spinal nerve cells pass] and
arthritis that limit a person's ability to walk any distance or
stand up straight. Often both problems can be corrected by
extending the fusion one vertebra lower.

Q: *Do you have to, in effect, start over with the fusion?*
A: Not at all. If you are adding one level to the fusion, all you do is
remove the old hardware and then, using a series of hooks,

latch on to the outer table of the old fusion mass and connect this to the anchor points in the additional vertebra to be added to the fusion. In fact, the technology is so good today that, occasionally, if the old hardware isn't in the surgeon's way and it's segmental enough, you can install a crosslink device and connect the new hardware to the old.

Q: *Do you ever have to fuse right down to the sacrum?*

A: I used to loathe fusing down to the sacrum—the non-healing rate was relatively high—but I don't have as many problems with that now because of advances in technology. Today, for example, if I do a one or two level addition of a fusion to the sacrum, I'll do a posterior fusion, but then I'll also do an anterior procedure. After I remove certain anterior discs, I put metal "cages" in the anterior disc space (along with bone graft). Then I insert pedicle screws and iliac wing screws, and connect them all up. If you try to do this operation from the back only, with no interdiscal devices, then your success rate is not likely to be good. By adding the concept of anterior column support, we have a very high success rate and a very happy group of patients because of the higher healing rate.

Q: *Is the removal of the discs always done anteriorly?*

A: Yes, most of the time. It makes the spine more correctible, and you can build in lumbar lordosis [the normal lower forward curvature of the spine] while you're at it. If the discs are removed from a posterior approach, the creation of more lordosis is not as easily achieved.

Q: *Do you usually prefer to do both the anterior and posterior procedures with lumbar revision surgery?*

A: Yes. Lumbar curves are generally such stiff curves that you wouldn't get enough correction by doing just a posterior procedure. Plus, if you're trying to fuse several levels, your fusion rate goes up enormously with front and back surgery. By adding the anterior part to the procedure, you end up with a bigger healing surface and a better healing rate. Both procedures help you move the spine into the position you want and you get a greater correction rate, so you've got the best of everything.

Q: *If a person is complaining of pain near the original instrumentation, what might you do?*

A: First, we determine what's causing the pain. If the problem is disc degeneration, fusion may be required. If the problem is prominent hardware, we either remove the instrumentation or alter it. If we discover an infection, we would explore the fusion mass, clean out the infection, remove the hardware, and subsequently administer antibiotics.

Q: *Is revision surgery an option for people who are older—say, in their seventies and beyond?*

A: Although I've had patients in their eighties with successful revisions, in general I try to avoid surgery on someone of that advanced an age. However, sometimes we consider it if a patient's problem is compromising his or her life, or if a patient has such a bad kyphosis or stenosis that he or she is just not really living. In these cases, though, patients must be willing to accept a much higher risk of complications, morbidity, or mortality.

Q: *What about older individuals whose problems cannot be safely dealt with by surgery? What do you do for them?*

A: We try to manage them medically and look at alternatives to surgery, such as pain management. For example, we may recommend long-acting or sustained-released narcotics or anti-inflammatories; these have probably done more to keep people functional and out of the operating room than anything else. We might also recommend cortisone, epidurals [injection of medication into the epidural space, the space surrounding the covering of a nerve root], nerve root blocks [the introduction of anti-inflammatory and anesthetic directly to an irritated nerve root], or facet blocks [the injection of an anesthetic into one or more facet joints of the spine]. One of our patients who was scheduled for a fusion to the sacrum opted for a series of facet blocks and epidurals. The blocks did such a nice job for her that she cancelled the surgery and went for two years relatively pain-free before finally deciding on surgery, which was ultimately successful.

Q: *Are there any other alternatives to revision surgery that you might recommend?*

A: The whole concept of mind-body medicine goes along with pain management. As a physician, I wouldn't rule out acupuncture or some of the Chinese-based holistic therapies. In fact, we work with an acupuncturist who seems to be successful in treating some of our patients. As far as I'm concerned, if you feel better after leaving the office of an acupuncturist or other alternative medical provider, there's nothing wrong with it.

Flat-Back Syndrome

Another potential reason for revision surgery is flat-back syndrome. To understand this problem, I asked Dr. Michael LaGrone, a spine specialist at the Texas Tech University Health Sciences Center in Amarillo, to talk about the syndrome and what can be done about it.

Q: *What is flat-back syndrome?*

A: Flat-back syndrome is a postural disorder caused by the loss of lumbar lordosis of the spine after one has scoliosis surgery. The normal lumbar curvature becomes flat, or you may even get a reverse curvature [called *lumbar kyphosis*]. The condition is characterized by the inability to stand up straight, and typically patients will have back pain in their upper or lower spine. It can occur in people of any age, but it is more likely to be found in older adults who have had scoliosis surgery.

Q: *What causes the condition?*

A: The most common cause is the use of distraction instrumentation, such as a Harrington rod, in the lumbar spine. Obviously, the patients who have the most severe flat-back syndrome are those who have had distraction instrumentation placed all the way down to the sacrum. Occasionally, we see patients who have *thoracolumbar kyphosis*—a deformity above the lumbar area that aggravates the forward positioning of the spine and causes flat-back syndrome. But far and away the most common causative factor is the use of distraction instrumentation in the lumbar spine.

Q: *What do spine surgeons do to prevent this problem?*

A: Most—but not all—spine surgeons know not to use distraction instrumentation in the lumbar spine. In the early days of scoliosis surgery, surgeons were more concerned with the frontal plane of the deformity and were not as aware of the sagittal, or lateral, plane, and over time they began to see patients with these problems. It soon became apparent that the sagittal plane was just as important as the frontal plane, and we realized the importance of not using distraction instrumentation in the lumbar spine. As a result, the incidence of flat-back syndrome has diminished, but we still see it.

In addition, we are very aware of the importance of maintaining the patient's lordosis during surgery. We do that by positioning patients with their hips extended so that we can preserve the lordosis while we are performing the surgery.

Q: *When would an individual realize he or she had flat-back syndrome? Immediately after surgery?*

A: Actually, the syndrome is usually noticed over a gradual period of time, and it can worsen. The distraction rod flattens the spine immediately, but some patients can compensate for this by extending the upper spine or hips. Over time, they can become more symptomatic—they may lean forward or they may lose hip flexibility. And if the fusion wasn't solid to begin with, they'll gradually lose even more of their lordosis.

Q: *What can be done about flat-back syndrome?*
A: Prevention is the key. Today we use segmental, instrumentation systems with multiple hooks, wires and pedicle screws that enable us to maintain the normal sagittal contours of the spine.

Q: *What should a person do if he or she has flat-back syndrome?*
A: The majority of those who have mild to moderate flat-back syndrome will probably be fine—they'll be able to keep their spine balanced by compensating for it above their fusion or below, and by keeping fit. It's difficult to predict whose flat-back will get worse, so it's a good idea to be monitored every year or so. If the condition is already severe, and the individual is unable to stand erect, that patient will probably be a candidate for surgical correction.

Q: *What is the surgical treatment for flat-back syndrome?*
A: Surgical treatment is very complex and the risk of complications is high. Typically, we do what are known as *closing wedge osteotomies:* We remove wedges of bone from the fusion mass and close the wedges down so that we can reestablish the lordotic curvature. Generally, patients do better and have a higher fusion rate if we precede the osteotomies with an anterior discectomy [disc removal] and fusion of the lumbar spine. Then we do our posterior osteotomies and use rigid segmental instrumentation to maintain the correction.

Q: *After surgery, what can patients expect?*
A: For older adults, I would probably recommend wearing a lightweight protective brace for six to nine months while the spine is

healing. For adolescents, a brace might not be needed if the internal fixation is rigid enough.

Q: *Do many people suffer from complications after the surgery to correct flat-back syndrome?*

A: In one of our studies, done in 1988, we found that 47 percent of fifty-five subjects continued to have some symptoms of leaning forward, and 36 percent continued to have moderate to severe back pain. Thankfully, our results are better today because of our increased knowledge and improved techniques.

Surveying the Risks of Scoliosis Surgery

Anyone who is having scoliosis surgery should be aware of the risks involved. To get an overview of the kinds of problems that may occur, I interviewed Dr. Oheneba Boachie-Adjei, Chief of Scoliosis Service at the Hospital for Special Surgery in New York.

Q: *Complications are possible with any type of surgery, but would you put the risks of spine surgery into perspective, starting with adolescents?*

A: In the majority of cases involving healthy adolescents with idiopathic curves from 45 to 70 degrees, more than 95 percent usually have very good outcomes. They will have a solid fusion whether treated from the front (anteriorly) or from the back (posteriorly), with instrumentation. These patients have a very low risk of developing infections, seldom have a problem with pain, rarely require medication after they leave the hospital, and can return to normal activities within six months to a year. This is true in my practice and in other clinics throughout the country. It is rare that such otherwise healthy individuals have in-

strumentation problems, and they do particularly well with
segmental fixation. In fact, in our practice, the incidence of
neurological problems such as paralysis is almost zero now. But
we still recognize the potential for these risks, monitor neurologic functioning, and perform wake-up tests on all patients.

Q: *What about the risks for adults?*

A: Adults with curves in the range of 45 to 80 degrees, particularly
those who have had a single-stage fusion, do very well in terms
of curve correction—averaging 50 percent. About 80 percent
get relief from pain, instrumentation-related problems are mini-
mal, the incidence of infection is low (less than 2 percent), and
neurological deficits, in my practice, are approaching the low
levels seen in adolescents, again with similar monitoring techniques.

Q: *What are the risks as patients age?*

A: As you approach the sixth and seventh decades of life, the statistics change. Nearly 50 percent of these individuals will experience problems including pseudoarthrosis (failure of the bone
to fuse), which can lead to loss of correction or implant failure.
Some experience wound healing problems or infection, heart
and lung difficulties, and problems with blood clots. The mortality rate is higher than in younger adults, but with improvement
in modern anesthetics and medical care, those older patients
are doing much better today. Proper patient selection and the
experience of the surgeon are of paramount importance. Due to
the poor quality of bone in older adults, instrumentation problems are more common than in young adults.

Q: *What can surgeons do during spine surgery to prevent neurologic
risks?*

A: To prevent risks of spinal-cord injury, we use electrodiagnostic
monitoring. One type helps us to monitor the posterior column,
or sensory pathway; another monitors the anterior column mo-

tor pathways. We always do a wake-up test during the surgery to make sure the patient has normal neurological function. On patients who have complex deformities who are at high risk for neurological problems, we do all three. We also are careful not to overcorrect a curve. We try to get the best balance and safest correction possible.

Q: *What else do surgeons do to reduce the possibility of complications?*
A: Another way to reduce risks when front and back procedures are required is to do both surgeries in one stage, under the same anesthetic, on the same day. In one of our reviews, we found that patients who had the surgeries at different times were more likely to become malnourished, had poorer wound healing, and experienced significant anxiety and pain while waiting for the second surgery. Of course, a two-stage procedure also requires a longer stay in the hospital and costs more, too. Other spine centers have had different results, but 90 percent of my adult patients who have front and back surgeries on the same day have done very well. However, in complex procedures for high-risk and medically unstable patients, a two-stage procedure is the best alternative.

Q: *Should patients ask their surgeons about the kinds of complications their patients have experienced as the result of spine surgery?*
A: I suppose so. Surgeons who have busy practices should have enough data to provide their patients with their complication rate. Doctors in a smaller practices probably don't have enough data to arrive at a rate, but they still should be able to discuss complications with published data across the board. If your surgeon has a small practice, you should ask about the reported complication rate to obtain some idea of what risks you face.

Q: *What do you tell your patients about risks before surgery?*
A: In our practice, we try to tell patients about positive outcomes, have them talk to other patients, and discuss with them all the

potential risks and benefits. We disclose problems we've had. We try to give them as much information as possible. We also encourage patients to bring family members along during this discussion.

Q: *What advice would you give the average person facing scoliosis surgery?*

A: Be aware of the treatment alternatives and the prognosis for your condition if untreated surgically. Most of all, try to be in the best physical condition you can. You should try to be in good nutritional shape—do not lose weight acutely unless you are obese—and if you smoke, you should stop. You should maintain good aerobic function and capacity, and exercise for strength and endurance. Read up on the literature, and prepare to be in a good frame of mind. Thinking positively is very important. Talk to other patients who have undergone procedures similar to the one you are facing. Of course everyone is different, but this will give you some idea of what is ahead.

Surgical Results: What Can You Expect?

It is vitally important for you and your doctor to have a clear picture—and a comparable understanding—of what surgery will do for you. If your expectations are unrealistic from the start, you will be dissatisfied with the results.

So what can you reasonably expect from surgery? To find out, I consulted with Dr. Michael Neuwirth, Director, Spine Institute, Beth Israel Medical Center in New York City. Here are excerpts from our discussion:

Q: *What can adolescents reasonably expect from scoliosis surgery?*

A: Since the primary objectives of surgery on adolescents are to arrest curve progression and prevent future problems, reasonable expectations include successful stabilization of the spine, safe correction of the deformity, a return to normal levels of activity as quickly as possible, and, after full healing, the ability to participate in all activities without restriction. Your surgeon will hope to fulfill all of these expectations. Safe correction of the deformity, however, does not mean *complete* correction. Even the most successful scoliosis surgery leaves patients with some degree of deformity.

Q: *What about expectations for adults?*

A: If you are an older adult who has an established, significant deformity *and pain,* the goals of surgery should also include relief from that pain as well as prevention of any further deterioration and increase in curve size. The ability to achieve pain relief through surgery, however, will vary depending on the type of curve and the specific causes of the pain. No matter how successfully the surgery turns out, an adult with lower back pain will not become completely pain-free. If things go well, the surgeon may significantly reduce your level of pain and allow you to function better, but you will probably always have some degree of back pain.

Q: *What is the biggest difference between surgeons' and patients' expectations regarding scoliosis surgery?*

A: The difference usually falls in the area of cosmetics. I believe the vast majority of adults who decide to undergo scoliosis surgery have at least some concern about their appearance, though their primary goal is generally the reduction of pain. Some teens considering surgery may not care about anything other than the reduction of their rib humps and the correction of their cosmetic deformities. If I stabilize these teenagers' backs and do not correct the cosmetic deformity that is their main concern, they will not be happy with the results. For children, the risk of continued curve progression and the likelihood of future pain may seem too remote to raise concern. Despite the importance attached to cosmetic correction by most children and adults who undergo scoliosis surgery, very few actually tell their surgeons that appearance is an important motivating factor for them.

Q: *What can patients expect with respect to correction?*

A: The amount of correction a surgeon can achieve through internal fixation and spinal fusion depends upon the age, and hence the flexibility, of the patient and on the surgical approach chosen. The amount of curve correction in teenagers and young adults typically ranges from 50 to 60 percent, while in adults the average is closer to 40 percent. Anterior surgery (operating on the front of the spine) can result in better correction, perhaps 70 to 80 percent in young people and around 50 percent in adults.

Q: *Can a surgeon accurately predict the degree of correction prior to surgery?*

A: A surgeon cannot tell you with any degree of certainty how much the curve will be corrected before he or she gets into the operating room. Only then will a surgeon make a decision about how much he or she can correct the curve comfortably and safely. Knowing how much to correct is done by experience and by feel. Through extensive experience, a scoliosis surgeon develops a feeling for what can and cannot be accomplished. That's why training, specialization, and experience form the criteria for a good scoliosis surgeon. In a young, flexible patient, surgery might bring a 50-degree curve down to 10 degrees if correction happens easily and without much stress or trauma. That's an 80 percent correction. On the other hand, if the curve is very stiff, the surgeon may be able only to bring a 50-degree curve down to 40 degrees—just a 20 percent correction.

Q: *Could a surgeon achieve 100 percent correction?*

A: That would be extremely rare. As scoliosis progresses, it changes the shape of the vertebrae themselves. This alteration in form makes it impossible to attain a perfectly straight spine through surgery. Another reason to avoid striving for 100 percent correction is the possibility of *overcorrection*. A person who has, for example, a right thoracic curve also often has smaller compensatory curves above and below the major curve. If the surgeon performs a selective thoracic fusion (that is, fusing only the vertebrae involved in the major curve) and overcorrects that curve, the compensatory curves may not adequately correct themselves in response to the overcorrection of the thoracic region—the patient may become *decompensated*. Finally and most important, as the forces applied to achieve correction increase, the risk of damage to the spine also rises. If a surgeon pushes too hard, he might fracture one or more vertebrae or even induce some neurological dysfunction. The serious risk of these complications discourages experienced surgeons from striving for perfect correction. Remember, the primary goal of scoliosis surgery is *not* total correction, but rather balance and compensation.

Q: *What steps should patients take to ensure they have realistic expectations?*

A: Talk to your surgeon about appropriate goals and expectations. Make sure you understand what the surgeon wants to accomplish, why he or she wants to accomplish that, and how he or she expects to do it. Just as important, make sure you let the surgeon know in detail, prior to surgery, what *your* expectations for surgery are, too, whether they seem obvious to you or not. Your doctor will be able to tell you how realistic those expectations are. If you and your surgeon share similar expectations, you will be much less likely to be disappointed by the surgical results and your surgeon.

No matter what your specific condition or the type of surgery recommended, I urge you to do your homework before you go ahead with it. And that means asking your surgeon some pointed questions, including the following:

- How many surgeries have you done?
- Which type of technique do you perform most often?
- How many of those do you do each month?
- May I have names and phone numbers of patients on whom you've performed this particular type of surgery?

You should be satisfied with the answers you get, discuss the surgery with your specialist, and understand all the risks that may be involved with your particular condition. If you do all that, you will be one step closer to a straighter spine and a lifetime of good health.

5

Undergoing Surgery

I f you and your doctor have agreed that you are going to go ahead with surgery, don't expect to be checked into the hospital the very next day. First, he or she will do a complete assessment of your spine. You will have x-rays taken in various positions: standing—front, back, and side—and bending. These will help your doctor determine how flexible your spine really is, how much he or she will be able to straighten it, and how many levels of the spine will have to be fused. X-rays also provide a graphic record of what your spine was like before surgery and help the doctor determine which procedure will be best for you.

Even if the x-rays reveal that you are a good candidate for surgery, you won't be packing your hospital bags just yet. Since scoliosis surgery is rarely performed on an emergency basis, it may be two or three months before you find yourself in the operating room.

For some people, this is an excruciatingly long period of time to wait. They just want to get it over with! Actually, this hiatus is a blessing in disguise because it gives you time to come to terms with the fact that you're really going to have surgery and to organize your life so that when the big day arrives, there aren't any niggling details hanging over your head or tasks left undone that could interfere with your complete recovery.

One of the first things to know is this: Even under the best of circumstances, the prospect of surgery is going to cause anxiety, so this is an especially good time to consider making use of a relaxation technique, such as meditation or muscle relaxation. Researchers have found that relaxation can be beneficial in lowering heart rate and blood pressure, boosting the immune system, and decreasing the amount of distress you feel.

Learn Relaxation Techniques

If you find yourself fretting about surgery in the days or weeks before it, you may want to try a simple technique to limit worry that was developed by Dr. Thomas D. Borkovec and his colleagues at Pennsylvania State University. This involves doing the following:

- Learn to identify worrisome thoughts that are unnecessary or unpleasant.
- Establish a half hour of "worry time" to take place at the same time and same place each day.
- If you find yourself worrying at various other times of the day, try to postpone the worry to that half hour you have scheduled as "worry time," and then try to get absorbed in other activities.

Other techniques, including meditation and progressive relaxation, can be learned with the help of a professional in these fields or from the many excellent books and audiotapes available on these subjects, and can be helpful both before and after surgery—or at any time, for that matter.

Contact Your Insurance Carrier

Having spine surgery is costly. Depending on where you have surgery performed, a one-stage procedure, plus a four- to five-day stay in the hospital, can cost upwards of $35,000; a two-stage procedure, with a stay in the hospital of up to seven days, can run $70,000 to $85,000—or more. Therefore, the first thing you should do is consult with your insurance agent to see whether the surgery and hospital stay will be covered by your policy. Most insurance companies, such as BlueCross BlueShield, have what is known as an 80/20 policy, which means that after you meet your deductible, the company will pay 80 percent of the surgeon's fee and 80 percent of the cost of the hospital room, and you are responsible for the remaining 20 percent. If you belong to a health maintenance organization (HMO), the company may pay 100 percent of the bill, but they will likely dictate your choice of doctor and hospital.

If you don't have insurance, it is wise to talk with your doctor (or your doctor's assistant) to find out if the hospital provides funds that can be used for patients with financial difficulties. Failing that, you may want to make arrangements with your bank to take out a loan.

Most insurance companies now require that you get a second opinion before undergoing surgery; they want to assure themselves that the procedure is required for medical, not cosmetic, reasons. Find out if your insurance policy has this requirement, and, if it does, you can ask your orthopedist to refer you to another qualified surgeon for evaluation.

Organize Personal Details

Once you have the financial details in order, you should begin the second phase of presurgical preparations—tying up the loose ends in your personal life. Talk with your teachers or your employer about the length of time you expect to be away. Your doctor can give you a pretty good estimate of this, based on the type of surgical procedure that will be done, and whether or not you need one operation or two. Also make sure that these individuals understand that spine surgery is *major* surgery—you won't have the strength or desire to slave over makeup work during your recuperation period. To be sure, there have been people who have had spine surgery and, because they were overachievers (or endowed with big reserves of adrenaline), have managed to overcome postsurgical fatigue and resume the activities of daily life. But for the majority of us, the healthiest way to regain strength after surgery comes from getting sufficient rest, doing any prescribed exercises, eating well-balanced meals, and seeking support from family and friends. Whatever you do, don't expend a lot of energy worrying about what you will be missing while you're away from school or work. It will all be there waiting for you when you return!

If you live alone, or if you know that you will be spending the better part of your at-home recuperation by yourself, it is a good idea to arrange to have friends or relatives drop in on you several times a day after you come home from the hospital. No, you're not going to be flat on your back. In fact, you'll probably be up and about for many hours each day. But you may not feel like making your own meals, and you probably will not want to be slogging away at chores. In fact, most surgeons today advise postoperative patients to avoid physical tasks—vacuuming, carrying laundry, mopping, bending into the car to get groceries, and so on—as well as contact sports. An additional note: If you have to wear a postsurgical brace, you may find that you feel dizzy when you remove it to take a shower. (Your blood pressure will drop when you remove it.) If that happens, it's comforting to know there is someone just outside the door or down the hall in case you need assistance.

In additional to the physical benefits, it is psychologically therapeutic to have someone around during your recovery period. Just having someone to talk with can go a long way toward making you feel better. Many people experience slight depression after surgery, not unlike the postpartum blues that strike many women after they have given birth. New mothers often feel as if they have lost some control over their lives, or that they will never get their strength back. The same is true of many people who have any kind of major surgery.

Of course, if you have to wear a postsurgical brace, you may feel frustrated that the "real you" will be under cover for the next several months. I found it particularly aggravating to come to grips with the fact that my snug-fitting clothes would be gathering dust for all that time. Had it not been for those daily visits from caring friends and relatives who were willing to listen to me whine every once in a while, I don't think I would have gotten through my recuperation as well as I did.

About a month before surgery, you may be asked to donate blood to be used during your surgery. You may not have to donate blood, however. It is often possible to recycle and cleanse a patient's own blood cells during surgery and return them to him or her throughout the procedure. In fact, if you insist on donating your own blood or that of a family member, the blood will still be eradicated or cleansed as if it were from the general population.

Several weeks in advance, get a good checkup from your local doctor, pediatrician, or internist—someone who knows your health history well. All too often, patients come into the hospital, having spent months waiting for the precious surgical date, only to find that they have high blood pressure, sugar in their urine, or other problems that could have been discovered and treated earlier. "There is such emotional stress getting geared up for surgery," notes Dr. Robert Winter, an orthopedic surgeon in Minneapolis, "that it can be catastrophic if the operation has to be canceled for problems like these."

Surgical patients should try to stay in good physical condition as well. Eat sensibly and, if you consume alcohol, keep it to a minimum. Talk with your doctor about whether you need to engage in a fitness or weight-reduction program. And if you smoke, quit immediately! According to Bettye Wright, an Associate Fellow of the Scoliosis Research Society who is also a registered nurse at Rochester Hills Orthopedics in Rochester, Michigan, "Research has shown that smoking affects the integrity of a fusion, and that's critical. Heavy smokers do not fuse as well as nonsmokers. For that reason, many surgeons won't do surgery on patients who continue to smoke because they know the outcome probably won't be successful. We ask our patients to quit smoking one to three months in advance of surgery, and remind them that they cannot smoke while the fusion is solidifying."

As your hospital date draws near, it's a good idea to make up a checklist of things to bring with you to the hospital. Pack a pair of comfortable slippers without heels, a pair of low-heeled walking shoes, your favorite bathrobe, plus personal grooming items such as your toothbrush, toothpaste, comb, and brush. If you feel you need to bring makeup, go ahead. But believe me, you won't feel much in the mood to "put on your face." After surgery, I didn't care what I looked like—even though I'd packed enough foundation, blusher, and lipstick for a month of makeovers!

You will be given a hospital gown to wear during the brief period of bed rest after surgery, so don't bother bringing your own pajamas. It will be far easier for the doctor and nurses to check on your incision if you're wearing the standard issue, "open in the back" gown. You may want to pack a comfortable warm-up suit, because once you're out of bed and taking daily walks in the hospital corridors, you may want something that doesn't look "medicinal." One week before surgery, make a special effort to get your rest. Dr. Winter advises that patients should arrive at the hospital rested, not exhausted.

Prior to your arrival at the hospital, your doctor will ask you to fill out various forms that the hospital will keep on file, including an *informed consent*. This important document says, in essence, that you and your doctor have discussed (and that you understand) the nature of your surgery, as well as its risks and possible complications.

Preadmission Testing

As much as a week before surgery, you'll go for preadmission testing (known universally as PAT) at the clinic or hospital outpatient department. There, staff members will perform an assessment, which includes a physical exam, x-rays, and a variety of tests. For example, the staff will check your blood pressure to make sure your blood will flow properly during surgery; they will also test your lung capacity to ensure that you are able to inhale and exhale properly. They will take samples of your blood and urine to make sure you don't have any sort of infection. They will weigh you and measure your height as well. (If you're having surgery at a hospital located out of state, many of these tests may have been done by your family doctor and forwarded to your surgeon's staff for review.)

During your PAT, you and your family may also receive detailed educational information about certain tasks. For example, your doctor may—or may not—request that you learn the technique for administering an enema that flushes waste from your system. And he or she may—or may not—ask your family members to learn how to do your own presurgical "scrub," which involves the use of a special cleanser followed by the application of an antibacterial lotion that stays on your skin and helps to fight off microorganisms that can cause infection. In many parts of the country today, the scrub is done in the operating room by staff just prior to your surgery.

Your presurgical staff will answer any questions you may have, including one of the most common: Can I have breakfast the morning of surgery? Their answer will be emphatic: NPO—*non per os,* which is Latin for "nothing by mouth." In other words, nothing to eat or drink after midnight the night before surgery. In fact, some spine centers recommend that patients not eat a heavy meal after 7:00 P.M. the night before surgery. You may, however, brush your teeth in the morning—just don't swallow any water!

You will also be advised to stop taking aspirin, ibuprofen (in Advil, Motrin, and other over-the-counter medications), or other nonsteroidal anti-inflammatory drugs (NSAIDs) starting ten days prior to surgery. NSAIDs have a tendency to thin the blood, which could potentially affect the speed with which your blood clots during and after the procedure. If you have diabetes, you will be asked to see a cardiologist or endocrinologist prior to surgery.

The Day of Surgery

Many hospitals require that you arrive at the hospital two to two-and-a-half hours prior to surgery. Pre-op is an extremely busy time! Your back will be scrubbed, and if you are having an anterior procedure, you may also need to be shaved. Blood may be drawn and you may need to provide urine for a urinalysis. In addition, a catheter will be gently placed into your urethra so that your urine can pass through it into a container. A spinal-cord monitor will be hooked up via sticky electrodes applied to the skin. At some point, a nurse will give you a sedative to make you drowsy. Most hospitals now do this intravenously—a needlelike tube, through which fluid is pumped, is inserted into a vein in your arm. Called an IV, it's slightly uncomfortable at first, but once in place (the tiny needle is secured by adhesive tape), you will hardly notice it's there. Soon, you will feel so drowsy so fast that if you try to count backward from ten to one, you will be asleep by the time you get to six or five. During this period, all of your lab reports will be reviewed by the doctor, nurse, and anesthesiologist.

Next you will be wheeled into the operating room, where a number of activities will be taking place—all without your knowing it, of course! First, if you are having a posterior procedure, you will be turned over onto your stomach and positioned on four "posters" that prop you up beneath your chest and hips so that you have plenty of breathing room. Your head will rest on a pillow that looks a bit like a donut; it's shaped this way so you have plenty of room to breathe. Your arms and legs will be positioned on other soft supports. In addition to the spinal-cord monitor, you will be hooked up to more devices: one that supervises your heart during surgery and another that can replace blood while the surgeon operates. Once these are in place, your anesthesiologist, who will sit by you during the entire operation, will place a breathing tube into your mouth or nose, through which you will breathe in the anesthetic, a sweet-smelling gas that will keep you asleep and oblivious to pain.

Most, if not all, doctors who perform scoliosis surgery use a technique known as the *Stagnara wake-up test* to monitor the spinal cord. During the operation, the patient is briefly brought to an appropriate level of consciousness and asked to wiggle his or her toes. Most patients will not remember that this extremely important test was performed.

Now the surgical team, having scrubbed up and donned their surgical gowns and masks, is ready to begin. Using a scalpel, your surgeon will make what is called a *midline incision,* drawn in a straight line despite the fact your back is curved. The length of the incision will depend, of course, upon the length of your curve(s). The surgeon and his or her team will then straighten your curve, using one of the multiple segmental techniques commonly used today. As you learned in Chapter 4, they will fasten multiple hooks and rods to your vertebrae, and place small chips of bone along your newly straightened spine that will fuse to it and create a solid mass of bone. Remember, by the time your spine heals, the hardware will no longer serve any function, but it will remain inside you for the rest of your life. To take it out would mean another surgery, and who would want that?

After the surgeon takes x-rays to ensure that all the instrumentation is securely in place, he or she will close up various levels of internal tissue with dissolvable sutures. For the external incision, the surgeon will probably use removable stainless-steel staples or pieces of Steri-Strip tape. Either of these closure mechanisms prevents the formation of a "railroad-track" sort of scar. In fact, by the time you heal, your scar will be just a fine line. (Mine is hardly visible, unless you're really looking for it.) In the small open space along the incision, the surgeon will insert a tiny Hemovac tube, which helps drain out excess blood and other body fluid that may accumulate.

Now the surgical team will remove the heart monitor and blood transfusion device, then gently turn you on your back. A nurse will wheel you (and your IV, and, if necessary, the spinal-cord monitor) to a postanesthesia care unit, where you will spend some time. You will still be in a deep sleep, however, so you won't be aware that nurses are still monitoring your blood pressure. In addition, your IV will now be pumping antibiotics into your system; this is necessary so that your body can fight off any infection that might occur.

After Surgery

Once you pass postoperative inspection, you will most likely be taken to your room. At some point thereafter, the nurses will remove your Hemovac tube, catheter, and any remaining monitoring devices. Because the anesthesia will begin to wear off now, this is a time of complete bed rest— you'll be flat on your back and asked not to raise your head beyond 30 degrees so that you don't put any pressure on your spine. Later on, two nurses will "log roll" your body every so often. Using a bedsheet for leverage, they will gently roll your body first to one side, then to the other. This technique prevents bedsores and keeps you from getting stiff. It also enables the nurses to easily view your incision and dressings.

Because your lungs were "relaxed" during surgery, they will now need to get a little exercise, so every four hours or so you will be asked to blow into an instrument called an *inspirometer* for as long as you are able. This also helps push out any mucus that might have accumulated during surgery, a situation that can sometimes lead to pneumonia. Many people find these "blow-bottle" exercises extremely difficult; these individuals are just so tired and weak that they don't want to do much besides rest. But do your best to puff away as often as you are asked to. Once you put your mind to it, you'll be surprised to learn how much lung power you really have!

During these two days of post-op observation, you will be allowed to have visitors, but only for brief periods. Most nurses are pretty flexible about extending visits, but, believe me, you're probably not going to feel much like schmoozing with parents or pals for more than ten or fifteen minutes at a time. You're still going to feel groggy; it can take anywhere from twenty-four to forty-eight hours to completely recover from the effects of anesthesia.

On day three, if not earlier, you will be moved to a special section of the hospital reserved for scoliosis patients. You will still have the antibiotic IV attached to your arm, and your nurse will have added a pain medication to the fluid. Much as I would like to say that undergoing scoliosis surgery doesn't hurt, I have to be honest. It does hurt. But thanks to the pain medication, these periods of discomfort can be managed. Today, pain medication is delivered via a system called *patient-controlled analgesia (PCA)*. Although the doctor determines the total amount and frequency of pain medication, this system allows the patient to push a button to get immediate relief from pain when it becomes necessary. Typically, a patient is allowed one-half grain of morphine every six minutes, and that's all he or she will get regardless of how many times she pushes the button. A word of caution from nurse Bettye Wright: "No one other than the patient should push the button. That means parents and visitors should not tamper with the delivery of pain medication under any circumstances."

Eventually, your IV will be removed. You can always ask for an occasional pain pill if you need it. When your appetite has returned a little and your stomach starts making "bowel sounds" (an indication that your intestines are working again), you will begin a progressive diet, starting with clear liquids and then moving first to full liquids, then to soft foods, and finally to regular food.

Depending upon the type of surgery you have had, you may be up and walking within forty-eight hours or so after surgery. Says nurse Wright:

Ideally, we like to get patients moving on the first day, but it doesn't always happen. If we can get them to dangle their feet over the side of the bed, that's wonderful. On the second day we want them at least standing and taking steps. Research shows that early mobility is very important to a rapid recovery.

This quick recovery time absolutely amazes me—when I had my first surgery back in 1970, I spent nearly two weeks afterward flat on my back! You will probably feel weak and a little wobbly when you first get out of bed. That's perfectly natural and nothing to worry about—you'll be getting stronger with each passing day. These first walks are never long and arduous—just five or ten minutes up and down the hallway—and in some ways they're fun; you're taking the first steps toward a successful recovery, and the new friends you've made in the hospital will be cheering you on! During the final days of your hospital stay—days five to seven for a single-stage procedure—you will continue alternating rest with daily walks to help you build up your strength.

If you are going to wear a postsurgical brace, you probably will have already been fitted for it prior to surgery. But because the contours of your back will have changed after surgery, your orthotist will return at some point after your surgery to double-check the measurements. You will likely be assigned to a physical therapist who will help you practice doing things in the brace. For example, to avoid the tendency to lean back in your brace while navigating on stairs, your therapist will teach you how to push yourself forward so that you don't lose your balance. You will also learn how to bend at the knees when you have to retrieve something from the floor. Most brace-wearers feel clumsy at first, but in time, they master the basics of daily life with ease.

Recuperating at Home

For the first four to six weeks after surgery, you should get as much rest as you need, but you should also increase your daily walks. They are essential to the healing process. In fact, studies have shown that the more physical conditioning you get after surgery, the faster you heal. But remember, walking is best; refrain from those "no pain/no gain" workouts! Also avoid excessive bending and twisting for any reason, and do not lift heavy objects. Keep in mind that it takes four to six months for an adolescent's fusion to heal, and six to twelve months for an adult's.

Within a week or so after surgery, you will no doubt visit your doctor. He or she will check your incision and your overall health, and take a standing x-ray to check on your correction. For most patients, the standing x-ray is be repeated at one month, three months, six months, one year, three years, and five years, and thereafter at the doctor's discretion.

Because the body uses a lot of energy to heal itself, you should increase your caloric intake during the recovery period, or longer if your doctor advises it. Don't worry about becoming a "blimp." Your body will be burning off the extra calories while it's mending.

About two weeks after surgery, adolescents usually can return to school. Adults may need anywhere from four to eight weeks or more to gain enough strength to return to work. In most cases, both youngsters and adults can resume activities that were a part of life before surgery, except for rough contact sports such as football. With your doctor's permission you may be able to swim (without the brace, if you have one) for a couple of hours a week. Each case is different, however, so make sure you talk with your doctor before engaging in any sports activities.

What about sexual activity during the recuperative period? Although you should talk with your doctor about your particular condition and how sex might affect it, generally speaking, it's perfectly all right to engage in sexual intercourse while you are recuperating—as long as, if you're a woman, you're using an effective means of birth control. Orthopedic surgeon Dr. Robert Winter advises that, with modern internal fixation techniques and good postoperative support, sexual activity can continue and there is no reason to avoid it for fear of upsetting the operative procedures. If you have been instructed to wear a postoperative brace, make sure to keep it on during sexual activity. Sometimes the margin of the brace can be irritating to the partner. If so, the edges can be padded. Acrobatic positions during intercourse should be avoided. The person who has had the surgery should, in most cases, take the less active role during intercourse.

About four to six weeks after surgery, you'll return to the clinic or hospital for x-rays. These will show your doctor (and you—if you want to see them) that your instrumentation is firmly in place and doing its job of correcting your curve. You will return several months later for more x-rays. By this time, those tiny bone chips used for grafting should have knitted together to form a solid bone mass. If they have, your doctor will probably give you permission to remove the brace—if one was required—for several hours each day so that you can swim or do other types of prescribed exercises. Your doctor will also be able to give you a rough idea of when you can remove the brace forever.

By the time you're free of the brace, you'll be back to normal. You will be as active as ever, and you will feel better than you ever did before surgery. Because your curve has been straightened out, you will be taller now—anywhere from one to four inches or more! Your clothes will fit better, too; shoulders, waistlines, and hemlines will be straighter, and if you had a rib hump before surgery, you can expect that it will be less noticeable—or that it has disappeared altogether!

What Do Patients Say About Spine Surgery?

Whenever I meet someone who is faced with the prospect of having spine surgery, I can usually predict that he or she will ask one or more of the following questions: "What's it like to have surgery?" "Does it hurt?" "How will I feel afterward?" "Will I be glad I had it done, or will I regret it?" In this section, you will get answers to those and other questions. You will meet youngsters and adults who have had operations to correct their scoliosis and who can tell you about their surgical experiences in their own words.

An Emotional Roller-Coaster Ride

Jennie L. learned she had a 25-degree scoliotic curve at age ten and wore a low-profile brace for five years. Unfortunately, her curve was a particularly stubborn one, and she had to have surgery on a 59-degree curve at age fifteen. As Jennie, now seventeen, recalls the details of her ordeal, it becomes clear it was an emotional roller-coaster ride for the entire family:

I was very scared about having surgery. I knew they were going to fuse my spine, and to me that meant I wouldn't be able to bend over, or that I'd walk like a robot or be a cripple. None of that happened, but I just kept thinking of the negatives and wishing they'd find some miracle drug so I wouldn't have to go through with it. In fact, when the doctor told me I'd have to have surgery, I flatly refused and said, "Nope, that's not gonna happen." I was crying the whole time, and he just kept saying that if I didn't have the surgery maybe I would be a cripple someday! My mom and I were so upset we just walked out on him. We knew he wasn't the doctor for us.

We did some research that confirmed I really should have surgery, so we met with many doctors until we found one we really liked. I had the surgery and was in the hospital for seven days. I don't remember much about the first two and a half days because I was on drip morphine for pain, but I kept asking my mom to read the same story over and over again. I don't know why, I just really wanted to hear that story! After that, I felt really sore, like I had a huge charley horse in my back muscles.

Some cool things happened while I was in the hospital. For example, a friend of mine acted like a coordinator to organize which friends could visit when. He made all the phone calls and planned when people should show up. Another friend made a big poster of pictures of me and my friends at birthdays and parties and band activities. Most of all, my friends just kept telling me, "You know, you're going to be all right. You're going to be normal." That helped a lot.

I think I've grown as a person since having the surgery. I saw and felt the worst during that time, but I got through it. I try not to let petty things upset me and now I can just brush things off. It was so hard to deal with everything leading up to the surgery, other things seem insignificant compared to it. It just made me stronger.

Jennie's mother, Carol, sees the details of her daughter's scoliosis from a different perspective. A self-described "Wonder Mom," she says that making the decision for her daughter to have surgery was one of the hardest things she's ever gone through. Here's why:

I'll never forget the day that we were trying on bathing suits before Jennie went to summer camp, and when she turned around to ask what I thought of one suit, I almost fainted! I just could not believe how much worse her curve had gotten in six months. I thought, "Oh my God, it's really bad." It flipped my stomach upside down!

No one in my family has ever had a medical issue to deal with, and I was one of those parents who said, "Anyone that lets someone put a metal rod in your child's back is crazy!" So when it came to deciding about the surgery, I had a lot of growing up to do.

We did a lot of research. We used the Internet and corresponded with other parents going through the same thing. It was a great tool for us, but I have to say to others: If you surf the Internet, be careful; there are a lot of horror stories out there, and it's difficult to determine what's true versus what is fabrication or exaggeration.

Finally, we found the right doctor. He was the only one who actually spoke to Jennie as a person, not just as a spine. My thoughts were, "This is not just your patient, this is my child. I need to know she's in good hands." If you don't like or trust your doctor, find someone else.

One of the many things I learned is that no matter how much you prepare for surgery, it never works according to the book. For example, we had read that a chest tube (for fluid drainage) would be in place for three or four days. So we were worried when Jennie needed hers for seven days. We later learned that it's not unusual to have it in place for eight to nine days; it just depends on the patient and the circumstances. We'd also read that the removal of bone graft from the hip is uncomfortable, but Jennie didn't have one day of complaint about that. Moreover, some kids come out of surgery and their faces are so swollen you don't recognize them, but not always. That could put parents over the edge if they're not prepared for the possibility.

We started a local support group for scoliosis patients and their parents in our community. A few things we've done have been particularly helpful:

- With bracing, the biggest concern seems to be self-esteem. Kids think they're going to look and feel different, and that others will laugh and make fun of them. If a youngster is worried about being in a brace, we suggest that he or she bring it to school. We did this with Jennie and everyone got to touch it and ask questions.
- In some cases, we now take kids on a tour of the hospital where they'll have surgery. We go into a classroom setting and go through what's going to happen every step of the way—and show them the equipment in the operating room and so on. We try to help them get more comfortable with what's going to happen. This doesn't work with all kids, however; some are too young emotionally and they get overwhelmed.
- We recommend that kids keep a journal of their experiences in the hospital afterward. Jennie got more out of reading her journal than anything else because so much was fuzzy. It helps kids put into perspective everything that happens to them.

CHOOSING THE ENDOSCOPIC APPROACH

When her daughter was four years old, J.C.'s mother noticed that her back looked crooked. From age six to ten and a half, the C curve in J.C.'s spine progressed from 25 degrees to 50 degrees, in spite of nearly five years of special bracing. Knowing that J.C. would have to have surgery, the family started searching the Internet. What they found was a new surgical procedure that would minimize scarring, trauma, and recovery time. The technique also showed a good success rate to date. J.C.'s mother, Bethany, felt they had found the solution to their problem:

I didn't want my daughter to have a posterior and anterior surgery, as well as a large scar. I wanted something minimally invasive, and the endoscopic approach seemed to be it. The doctor had to go through her chest to do the front part of surgery, then reposition and operate on the back part of the spine. But this new procedure—called thoracoscopic anterior spinal instrumentation and fusion—*allowed him to make four small one-inch incisions, then use a thoracoscope through the small incisions to do the fusion on the front part of the spine. He then attached screws and a metal rod to the vertebrae using the thoracoscope, corrected the scoliosis, and was able to forego having to instrument the spine from the posterior approach.*

Although J.C. was nervous about the surgery and the long-term outcome, I think she was relieved because she wouldn't have to wear a brace anymore. She went into the hospital on a Wednesday, had the surgery on Thursday, and was released the following Wednesday. She did well, and after three weeks at home, returned to school for two weeks of half-days. The doctors took the curve down to 11 degrees. That was dramatic! She did have to wear a protective post-op brace for a few months and didn't like it, but compared with the original brace, this was nothing.

It's been a year since the surgery. She's in full, unrestricted physical education class and her curve has actually improved. She doesn't look so lopsided, she breathes better, and her scars are little tiny things. I feel the endoscopic approach was ultimately less traumatic for my child, and I'm definitely a believer in it.

A Young Pilot's Story

In her freshman year in high school, Carey L. began to notice that "things weren't right" with her body. Her shoulders didn't line up right, and when she bent over in front of a mirror, she could see the beginnings of a rib hump. So she did what a lot of youngsters do: she camouflaged her crooked spine with baggy clothes. Eventually, her family doctor took an x-ray of her spine and discovered it was a double S curve. The top curve was nearly 60 degrees, the bottom, around 40 degrees. Carey describes the experience:

> *We were all sort of in shock. My mom burst into tears, and, I have to ad-mit, it was pretty traumatic to see the x-rays and how big the curve really was! I was not a very happy camper that day. The doctor's reaction wasn't comforting at all. He said surgery would be required and he knew a specialist. My folks were feeling really guilty because we never did anything when we first noticed I was crooked. Still, there was never a time when I thought, "I'm not going to do this." I wanted it fixed at any cost. Of course, I weighed the pros and cons, but it just didn't seem like something I had a choice about. My mindset was, "This is some-thing I am going to do." I had just gotten my private pilot's license and was thinking about becoming a pilot, like my dad. I didn't want to jeop-ardize that.*
>
> *Four months later, at age seventeen, I had the surgery, a six-hour pos-terior procedure. I have to admit I was pretty naive about it. I really went into it blindly, not knowing what the doctor was going to do or what it would be like afterward. All in all, I was pretty calm the morn-ing of surgery, but my family was so concerned, they were making me nervous. I was feeling, "Just wheel me off to the operating room!"*
>
> *That was ten years ago. As I look back on it, I wish I'd asked for step-by-step information about what was going to happen before, during, and after the surgery. As I said, I was pretty clueless. I also wish I had gotten a better result. Although the doctor was able to straighten the bottom of the curve, the top is still around 50 degrees, so my shoulders*

still look a bit uneven. Also, one of my rods irritates me. I'm not in pain at all, but I can definitely feel the rod every so often. That didn't stop me from getting a job as a pilot with a major airline, and I'm very happy with my life now. I'm glad I went through with it, although I definitely wish I'd gotten a better result.

PREPARATION IS THE KEY

Lori A. was diagnosed with scoliosis at age sixteen, but didn't have surgery until last year, when she turned forty-two. Her curve was slow to progress, but when it eventually reached 47 degrees, she believed it would continue to get worse and cause serious problems. She was concerned that she would have pain in the future and figured that surgery would go more smoothly in her forties than, say, in her fifties or sixties:

As I decided whether or not to have surgery, I considered several factors. First, my mother has osteoporosis, and I have several risk factors for it and was then premenopausal, so I figured it would be best to get it over with while my bones were still strong. Second, I was between jobs, and that seemed like a perfect time to have it done. Third, after many hassles with my insurance company, I learned that my plan would provide 100 percent of the hospitalization cost if I opted for surgery. Everything seemed to be in place.

I know I'm unusual in that I didn't worry very much about the actual surgery. I mean, I figured I'd be asleep! Also, I made a point of getting in shape before the surgery. My surgeon told me to strengthen my quads and upper body as well, since you do a lot of squatting when you're recuperating because you can't really bend over. So I went to the gym three or four times a week, used the treadmill and the stationary bike and weight-training devices. I think that help me recuperate relatively fast for my age.

I was in the hospital for eleven days. My lungs collected a lot of fluid, which I had to cough up—ouch!—so I had to have a bronchoscopy— double ouch! I also had terrible constipation due to the pain medica-

tions, but eventually that cleared up. I can't say that I ever felt any pain in my spine after the surgery, just discomfort and aching in my whole mid-area and on the right side of my back where they did the thoracoplasty to reduce my rib hump. For many weeks after surgery, if I had to sneeze or cough, I had to hold myself very tight!

I am now essentially straight and thrilled. In fact, I was so happy with my outcome and my hospital experience and the doctors and nurses, I've gotten a job as an administrator at an orthopedics institute. I didn't get any taller as a result of the surgery—that's something a lot of people want. With my anterior procedure, they took disks out, so any height I would have gained from straightening the curve, I lost with removal of the disks. But I'm already five-feet-eight, so I'm all right!

Tough Recuperation, but Relatively Pain-Free and Straight

Linda R. was 30 when her chiropractor took x-rays and noted that she had scoliosis. On the chiropractor's advice, she continued her weekly chiropractic treatments for the next year, but her curve continued to worsen. Moreover, because some of her discs had begun to deteriorate, she began to experience severe pain in her neck and lumbar spine. She quit seeing the chiropractor and sought the help of three different physical therapists, an acupuncturist, and a rheumatologist—anything she could think of to get herself out of pain:

When the pain started affecting my life, I figured it was time to think about surgery. It was hard to stand or walk for any period of time, and although I'd always been active, I wasn't able to hike or go for long walks—the pain was excruciating and I didn't like feeling disabled! So I met with an orthopedist, told him I wanted to put off the surgery for a year, and he put me in a low-profile TLSO [thoracic-lumbar-sacral orthosis] brace that I wore for short periods of time. I only wore it if I was going to walk or stand for a long time, but it really did work.

I planned my surgery nearly ten months in advance so that I could get my business in order; I chose to have my surgery at the low point of my workload. I had plenty of time to get in shape as well, which I knew would be important for recovery from such a big surgery.

I wasn't afraid of the surgery in the beginning. Everybody seemed to say, "Oh everything's great and in three months you're out of pain and everything will be great." But then I started really digging, really talking to people. That's when I started hearing that it's a pretty damned painful surgery and recovery is tough. When I started hearing that, the prospect of surgery became harder to think about. I don't think people wanted to scare me. It's just that they sugar-coated or underreported their experiences.

I had both the anterior and posterior surgery on the same day, and I had a tough time of it. I was in the hospital for twelve days, five of them in intensive care because I had breathing problems. That's why I always tell people now to expect the unexpected with surgery! I certainly didn't expect to wake up and be breathing through a tube.

There's nothing that can describe the way you feel after surgery, and everybody's different. My back felt heavy. It was the toughest period I've ever gone through as an adult. But remember, I was forty-two when I had the surgery. Kids do much better than adults. And I've actually talked with women in their seventies, and I'm amazed they do as well as they do, considering what I went through.

Despite my difficulties, including shoulder-blade pain because they had to fuse in the cervical area, I absolutely feel better for it all. The first time I stood up after surgery, I thought, "This is completely different." The lumbar pain was entirely gone. By the time I was a year post-op, I had resumed all the activities I'd had to give up—hiking, museums, and parties. That in and of itself made it worthwhile because I'm such an active person. I'm really surprised at how flexible I am, though you don't want to see me putting on pantyhose because that's a joke! My shoulders are completely level now. My life is back to normal, and I've got a damned straight spine!

A Positive Attitude Ensured Success

Randy P. is one of many people who wish they had had scoliosis surgery a lot sooner than they did. Although he was diagnosed as having scoliosis at the age of thirteen, it was not until he turned twenty-two that he finally checked in to the hospital to have it corrected. Unlike many people I interviewed, Randy did not ignore his curve during those intervening years. Far from it! He wore a Milwaukee brace night and day for five whole years—but unfortunately, as sometimes happens, his stubborn curve refused to respond to it. He recounts:

> In seventh grade, when my mom and I noticed that my rib cage was twisted a little, we went to our family doctor. He took x-rays, and we learned that I had a slight curve of about 10 degrees. He said it probably was nothing to worry about, but suggested we see a doctor at a scoliosis clinic, just to be on the safe side. By the time we got around to making the appointment—about two months later—my curve had progressed to 25 degrees. It was just racing out of control! I wasn't in any kind of pain, and my rib cage didn't really look worse, but we couldn't ignore what the x-rays were saying.
>
> So they put me in a Milwaukee brace, neck ring and all. Needless to say, my reaction was very negative. I didn't want to go back to school, and I had a lot of trouble getting clothing to fit over it. No matter how much padding there is on braces, they just eat up your clothes. I never bought a decent shirt the whole time I had to wear my brace.
>
> I wore that thing twenty-three hours a day, every day, but each time I went back for a checkup, my curve was 5 to 10 degrees worse. By the time I reached twelfth grade, it had progressed into the high 40s. But because of my age, the doctors felt that I'd matured enough so that it would slow down or stop at that point. So they finally took me out of the brace, and we all agreed that I'd keep coming back for checkups from time to time.
>
> I kept going back to the clinic while I was in college, and, sure enough, it got worse. Finally, when the curve had reached 62 degrees, the doctors told me that I couldn't put off surgery any longer. They were

worried that the curve might cause some spinal-cord damage. And by now, my body had changed quite a bit—although I didn't have a rib hump, my chest and shoulders were so uneven, it looked like my body was twisted half over to the other side.

My first reaction was, "Well, I knew this was coming," because it had kept on getting worse over the last four or five years. But my second reaction was one of bitterness—why did I have to spend all those years in the brace when it didn't seem to have done me a whole heck of a lot of good?

I was pretty frustrated about it, because I've also had a lot of medical problems ever since I was little—none of them little picky things, either. I was born with a cleft lip and cleft palate, and had to have major surgery to correct those. And since those problems caused a severe underbite, and because my teeth were all over the place in my mouth, I had to have more surgery to move my front jaw out about an inch and a half, then had to have my mouth wired shut for a month. By themselves, those surgeries wouldn't have been so bad, but I was in the Milwaukee brace at the time I had them done! Still, I'm a pretty tough bird most of the time, and I really have never let that kind of crap get me down. But believe me, there have been days when I've felt, "God, just to be average!"

Maybe because I'd gone through other types of surgery, I wasn't that upset about having scoliosis surgery. Of course, I was going through finals week at college, so I didn't really have much time to think about it.

The night before I had surgery, the doctor came in and explained that he was going to do a Cotrel-Dubousset technique on me—he'd fuse eight of my vertebrae and then put in two rods with wires. He did say he might wind up doing something different once he got in there because they often don't know for sure which technique to use until they actually see your spine. But at that point, he was pretty sure he'd do the C-D, and that meant I probably wouldn't have to wear a brace after surgery. As a person who'd already spent five years cooped up in a brace, I was relieved to hear this—in fact, that's probably the only reason I didn't cut out of the hospital and go home that night! I'd seriously considered just sneaking out and getting on a bus and going home—nobody would have known where to find me!

I really got a lot of psychological support from the nurses. Many of them had had scoliosis surgery themselves. When I asked one of them, who had become pregnant many months after her surgery, whether having a steel rod in her back was hard on her, she said, "No, I hardly notice it at all." Just hearing that made me feel a whole lot better.

I wasn't too nervous the night before surgery, but in the morning, that was a different story. I was real nervous then. But my mom and dad were there, and that helped a lot. Both of them have had surgery for disc problems, so we all talked about our feelings. It was nice to know that they could personally understand what I was going through.

I wasn't too worried about the pain after surgery—I've done a lot of hurting in one way or another in my life. But when the anesthesia wore off, it felt as if a Mack truck had run over my back—literally! Let me tell you, I don't cry very often, but that was quite a night! I was only in really bad pain for about a half an hour, though, because they gave me medication. Don't get me wrong. It still hurt, but it wasn't unbearable.

I'm the kind of person who doesn't let things slow me down, so the day after surgery, I was out of bed walking around. I got out of the hospital about seven days later and didn't have much trouble at all. I did a lot of sleeping and lying around, but I never got depressed—I don't let stuff like that get me down too much.

About three and a half weeks after surgery, I was back into the swing of things. I had to take it a little easy at school—I couldn't carry the twenty pounds of books I used to lug around with me—and I did get tired a lot. But overall, surgery hasn't slowed me down hardly at all.

Although my curve was corrected to about 30 degrees, I'm still a little crooked, but basically, I'm much better. My shoulders are much more even now, and so is my chest. And even though I didn't have any cardiopulmonary problems, I think I'm breathing better now. To me, the surgery was well worth it.

Anybody who's going to have surgery needs to hang tough, I think. It'll be rough for a while, but in the long run, it's better to go through with it because you can take all the pain in a week's time, and then not have the problems for the rest of your life. Or you can do nothing and have real serious problems forever. The aftereffects of surgery can be hard to live with, but the only thing that can really slow you down is

your own attitude about it. If you've got a good, positive attitude about
surgery, it really doesn't slow you down much at all.

A FANTASTIC SHAPE

Although Maria H., now fifty-two, knew she had scoliosis at the age of
thirteen, she spent many years ignoring her curve—until it had progressed
to 84 degrees. By that time, although her lumbar curve was not terribly noticeable—she could conceal it with the "right" clothes—there was no ignoring the pain. Still, it was not until four years later that she finally had
surgery, and, as you will see, the anxiety she suffered in the intervening
years was more than most people deal with in a lifetime. Happily for
Maria, however, the ordeal was worth it:

> *I suffered for many years from the scoliosis in my back, but I really*
> *didn't know anything could be done about it. I kept fooling myself that*
> *it wasn't getting worse. I kept eliminating activities from my life so that*
> *I'd have less pain, and sometimes I could convince myself that the pain*
> *had decreased, but it really hadn't—I was just doing a lot less.*
>
> *All the doctors I went to in America and in Germany, where I once*
> *lived, said nothing could be done for me. No one ever mentioned that*
> *surgery was available. I'm amazed that no doctor ever even hinted to me*
> *about it. So I kept looking around for books and articles on the subject,*
> *and finally, in a book about general health, I found a section about sco-*
> *liosis, and that's the first time I ever knew there was such a thing as Har-*
> *rington rod surgery.*
>
> *That gave me a little hope, so I went to an orthopedic surgeon in At-*
> *lanta to see whether anything could be done. I told him I had a lot of*
> *pain, and he took an x-ray of my spine that showed my curve was 84 de-*
> *grees. He said he couldn't do a thing except give me exercises to do! I*
> *couldn't believe it! I said to him, "I have so much pain and you tell me*
> *there is nothing you can do?" As I said this, he was instructing his nurse*
> *to give me information about the exercises and was about to leave the*
> *room when I said, "What about surgery and the Harrington rod?"*

His eyes lit up and he said, "You mean you'd be interested in something like that?" I said that I would, and he gave me the name of a spine specialist.

When I met with the new surgeon, I wasn't convinced that I should have the surgery. It seemed scary and frightening to me, and the surgeon seemed cold and unfeeling toward me. I didn't trust him, didn't get a good feeling about him, so I decided that I would just continue to try and live with the pain.

That didn't work, and I eventually found another surgeon in another state. He took x-rays of my spine and told me that I must have surgery and that I should not wait any longer. But then he showed me an x-ray of another patient who had had surgery and it looked terrible and shocking to me. I thought, "No, I'll never have this done to me." He did, however, give me the name of another orthopedist. I agreed to meet with him, but I knew in my heart I probably couldn't go through with it.

When I met the new doctor, he took x-rays of my spine. My curve had progressed to 87 degrees. Of course, he recommended that I have surgery, and by now I knew he was right. The whole atmosphere at the center was good and comforting—I knew it was the right place.

At first, I thought I'd only have to have one surgery. But after doing a lot of tests, the doctor told me that because many of my discs were destroyed due to the scoliosis, he would have to do two surgeries and fuse my spine all the way down to my hips! That really scared me, but he said it wouldn't make much difference in my life, that I could still do all the same things I'd done before. It took me a while to accept this, but I knew I would be in good hands. Thankfully, I had done a lot of research beforehand—all that information helped me judge for myself.

The night before surgery, I felt very positive. I blocked out any fearful thoughts from my mind. I had made up my mind that this was it. I knew my surgeon was an expert, and the rest would be up to Somebody Up There. Of course, my husband spent a lot of time with me at the hospital. He was very supportive and that helped a lot. But I knew most of it was up to me.

After the first surgery, I felt very much at peace and that everything was going to be just fine. I did have some pain, but a different kind than I had felt before. Your body is just in an upheaval after surgery, but luckily, I was mentally prepared for it so it wasn't that bad. I think you get mentally strong when you know you're going to have surgery. I got through the first surgery fine, so I believed the second one would be all right, too.

Ten days after the final surgery, I left the hospital to go back home. I felt fine, but I was afraid of having to take all those taxis to and from the airport, and to get on the plane. It was quite an undertaking, but luckily, I was able to lie down in the plane and rest, and I continued taking my pain pills. I did much better than I ever imagined!

When I got home, I kept thinking that the pain would never stop. When I would lie down, I felt good, but as soon as I'd get up, I got this indescribable pain—sort of like somebody pressing a big shoe in your back. But then, all of a sudden, the pain was just gone. It didn't fade away; it just disappeared. And within six weeks after the last surgery, I felt like my old self again. I continued wearing my brace for nine months, though I took it off for a while each day so that I could take a shower. And I also did a lot of walking—two miles a day!

My surgeon was right. I can do everything I did before, but now, instead of bending at the waist, I bend at the hips and come down with my knees a bit if I have to pick something up. It is no problem whatsoever, and I don't even notice it anymore.

I don't know how much my curve improved in degrees, and I didn't even ask. I'm not interested! I think I look perfectly straight compared to what I was before. And my scars are very nice—one starts on the side of my navel and goes around my hip upward to the back near my lower rib and the other is in the middle of my back. They both look good. I'm even going to a public swimming pool in a bathing suit—and that's something I would have never done before!

If I had known way back when what I know now, I'd have gone for surgery right away. It helps a lot to do your research, call anybody you can, read everything you can, and inform yourself before you go ahead with surgery. Then you make up your mind. I'm glad I did, because I'm in such fantastic shape now!

COMPLICATED BUT WORTH IT

Fifty-two-year-old Jane W. battled scoliosis nearly all her life. Diagnosed as having idiopathic scoliosis at the age of six, she spent the next several years wearing a corset and doing a variety of exercises. She was told these remedies would correct her curvature, but they didn't, and by the time she turned eleven, her curve had progressed to nearly 100 degrees. Not only did her S-shaped curvature create a huge rib hump on her back, it also squeezed her lungs so that her breathing capacity was only 35 percent of normal. Since that time, Jane has had four spine surgeries to correct her scoliosis, each one fraught with complications. But despite all the problems, she believes the surgeries were worth it. Today, when she looks in the mirror, she still remarks, "I can't believe it's me!"

Jane says:

Before I had my first two surgeries—spinal fusions done two weeks apart—I spent three months in the hospital bound up in a turnbuckle cast that covered most of my head and enveloped my body down to my knees. The cast was supposed to stretch me out a bit before I had the fusions. My parents and I went along with this because we believed that all these procedures would eventually get rid of my rib hump. But apparently we misunderstood the doctors—they don't always word things too well—because even after the surgeries, my hump was still there. The doctors told me there was no way of getting rid of it after all. As you can imagine, I was absolutely devastated!

Even though the fusions reduced my curve to 89 degrees, and the doctor told me my back was strong enough that I could be a hog carrier and that everything would be just fine, that didn't turn out to be true. Though I carried on with my life for many years, by the time I reached menopause, I started having respiratory problems. I coughed all the time and was so short of breath that just walking from the parking lot to the hospital where I worked left me gasping. So I had x-rays taken and learned that, despite the fusions, my curve had increased to 110 degrees!

Eventually, I went to another hospital and the doctor said he could fix my spine by doing two more surgeries—an anterior and a posterior. I was frightened, but I knew I had to do something. I didn't want to spend the rest of my life as a respiratory cripple.

I had to wait for three months before the hospital could take me, and even in that short period of time, my curve increased from 110 to 116 degrees. But when I checked into the hospital, I was full of high hopes and not the least bit frightened. Three people who had had the same type of surgeries had written to me and said they were feeling and looking great, and I also prayed a lot and felt that I received signs that said, "Go ahead with the surgery . . . it'll be great!"

After the first surgery, well, you name the complication and I had it. I developed a pulmonary embolism, a blood clot on the lung. When you reach my age and you have lung complications to begin with on top of the surgery, it's no wonder this happened. Then I developed a bladder infection and a kidney stone (a problem I'd had before), and from all the medications I was taking—the iron pills and pain pills—I developed gastritis. My stomach blew up like I was six or seven months pregnant. Needless to say, they had to postpone the second surgery for a few weeks until all those problems cleared up.

I was scared to go back for the second procedure, but as I've always said, "If you're swimming and reach the middle of the lake, you have to keep on going to get to the other side." So of course I went ahead with it. But I was miserable for quite a while afterward. I was worried that I'd develop another clot (but didn't), and I was in quite a lot of pain. I hated even being touched!

My curve is now down to 85 degrees, and even though I still tire pretty easily and am not too crazy about having to wear this brace, I think I look terrific and I'm breathing very well.

When I used to look at myself from the front, I looked a little dumpy. One of my breasts looked crooked and so did my shoulders—I looked like a tube of toothpaste that had been squeezed together, with a great big hump on the back of it. But now that I've straightened out, I just can't believe it's me! Even friends who used to say that they never noticed my hump think I look wonderful now, even though I have the brace on!

For me, the surgeries were hell, but they were short-lived. If you compare that to a lifetime, it's worth it. What are a few months compared to years of agony that keeps getting worse? Even with all the complications, if I had it to do over again, I would. What the doctors did for me was unbelievable!

A GOOD MINDSET HELPS

Lisa G., twenty-five, is a tough cookie by just about anyone's standards. Lisa ignored the protests of her worried parents and scheduled herself for spine surgery. She claims the experience never caused her a bit of pain and attributes her phenomenal recovery to her belief in "mind over matter":

When I was thirteen, my school doctor noticed a curve in my back and sent notes with me to take home to my mother. But because I was heavily into gymnastics and didn't want anything to ruin that, I threw the notes in the garbage. I knew somebody who had scoliosis, and she had to wear a brace—I didn't want to have to do that! The thought of having to wear a brace really scared me.

Nobody in my family knew there was anything wrong, and because I wasn't feeling any pain or having any other symptoms, I just went through high school with sort of a la-di-da attitude. I didn't notice that my body was curving at all, so I figured that there really wasn't anything wrong.

After I graduated and got a full-time job and had to sit at a desk all day long, it finally hit me. I started having a lot of pain in the middle of my back and in my shoulder blades. I still looked okay, but I had the pain, so I went to see an orthopedist. He took x-rays and said my curve was about 42 degrees. But because I was seventeen and almost full-grown, he didn't recommend a brace. He said it probably wouldn't do me much good and suggested that we just watch it to see if it would progress. I wasn't upset at that point, knowing how much worse it had gotten. I had made my choice earlier, by throwing away all those notes from the school doctor, and now I knew that I was going to have to live with it. About a year later, I went to a specialist who said he could op-

erate on me. But because I wasn't having any trouble breathing and he said the curve wasn't that bad, we decided we'd just wait a while longer to see if it got worse.

When I turned nineteen, my curve seemed to get a lot worse. I couldn't breathe properly, and I'd get stuck in one position from sitting all day at work. To get relief from the pain, I'd have to come home every night and lie flat on my back. So I started thinking about surgery again, but my parents were very scared of the idea and didn't want me to have it done, so I waited two more years before I saw a specialist again.

By the time I was twenty-one, my hips were starting to hurt, and I felt as if I were shrinking. I didn't feel good anymore. I couldn't bend the way I did before, my waist was all bunched up, and my clothes were tight around one shoulder. But I knew some people who'd had scoliosis surgery—people with curves a lot worse than mine—and they'd come through it just fine. So I made an appointment with an orthopedic surgeon.

After he looked at my x-ray, which showed my curve had progressed to 45 degrees, he told me I should have the operation. I was relieved when he said that, because I was going to ask him if I could have the surgery even if he didn't feel I needed it yet. I knew then that the curve would probably keep progressing unless I did something about it, and I just figured, "Why not have it done now, while you're still young?" I really wanted to have it done, because I was freaked out that I thought I was shrinking.

A week before the surgery, I checked into the hospital and they put a plaster cast on me to stretch me out a bit. I was feeling really good about it, because I knew that from then on I was going to look and feel better.

I was never nervous about the surgery. Not one bit. That's because I had a tremendous amount of confidence in my doctor. When he explained the surgery to me, which involved a Harrington rod, he talked about it like it was an afternoon tea party for him, and I figured if it was like that for him, then I had nothing to fear. And the man has done so many operations, so I figured there was no reason for me to get upset.

When I woke up after surgery, I didn't feel any pain at all. Honestly, it didn't hurt, though my doctor tells me I'm an exception to the rule.

Maybe that's because I had worked out on weights for two years before the surgery—I was in really good physical condition. And afterward, I was very mobile; I could move from side to side, and I even handled my own bedpan all by myself.

Of course, I had a good mindset. I was determined to have a good recovery, and I didn't ever let myself think I was unhealthy—because I'm not unhealthy; I was just apparently born with a curvature of the spine, and that doesn't mean I'm unhealthy.

Although I wasn't supposed to, I got up out of bed the second day after surgery. I just had to go to the bathroom, and I was real tired of using that bedpan. So I got the nurses to help me to the bathroom, and I didn't feel faint or anything. By the seventh day after surgery, I'd gotten my brace and was taking twenty-minute walks on my own. As a matter of fact, before the nurse came into the room to take me down to the main floor so I could go home, I'd taken a shower and gotten dressed by myself.

Once I got home, about the only problem I had was getting out of deep, cushiony chairs. And because I had to wear a brace, my bed didn't feel too comfortable, and I often felt really warm during the night. But I never needed any help getting dressed, I never took any pain pills, and I didn't take one nap.

Today I can do everything that I did before. I'm just as flexible as ever, and I can still lift things, as long as I do it properly. And I think I look much better. My waist is a lot longer and slenderer than it was, and I got an inch and a half taller. From the side, my rear end and lower back look a little flatter than they used to because they had to fuse a little way down into my lumbar spine, and I can't say that I like the look. [See page 96 for a discussion of flat-back syndrome.] But I'm still much better than I was before. I know I made the right choice. I didn't have any problems at all, and that's because 50 percent of it was my having a good mental attitude and being strong and in good condition. The other 50 percent is that my doctor was so wonderful and good at what he does.

To me, the surgery did not hurt. I was not uncomfortable, and I really mean that. But it's all in your mental attitude—I believe my mind has total control over everything I do and feel. Sure, you can make it miserable—my roommate in the hospital showed me that. She wasn't happy with anything or comfortable with anything. But she didn't try to be happy or comfortable; she didn't try to feel better. She just lay there in her misery, and she loved it! She didn't like the post-surgical brace, but she didn't even try to like it, so that made it even worse. She had a very bad time of it, but I think it's because she had a bad attitude to begin with. To me, the surgery was easy, though I know not everybody feels that way. I was lucky. In two weeks, I was out of there and felt great! I had just made up my mind that it was going to be fine, and it really was!

Quick Recovery, "Wonderful" Results

Like many adults who have scoliosis, Carolee M., fifty-five, knew some-thing was wrong at an early age—in her case, at fourteen. But because she developed a curvature at a time when doctors were not particularly well informed about scoliosis, she "learned to live with it" for many years. Luckily, however, she never gave up trying to find a surgeon who would be willing to operate, and today this mother of three grown children is happy, healthy, and as she puts it, "straightened out."

Carolee says:

My mother first spotted my scoliosis when I was dressed up to be in a wedding. She noticed that the buttons weren't straight and that my shoulders were off. Because this was the era of the polio epidemic, when we went to a doctor shortly thereafter, he said he thought it might be caused by polio (though we're really not sure about that, even today). But since he didn't know how to prevent it from getting worse, he said the best thing to do was rest, and he wouldn't allow me to participate in any high school activities such as gym class.

Eventually, I found another doctor who sent me to a workshop for polio victims at the Sister Kenny Institute. I went there three times a week, where they'd hang my body from the ceiling from ropes, which was supposed to keep the curve flexible and to keep it from getting worse. I thought it was helping, but a few years later, when I had to go into the hospital to have my appendix removed, a doctor noticed the curve and said, "Gee, you really should have surgery for that." But when my parents called my family doctor and told him that, he advised against it, saying that if I had surgery, I'd end up in a wheelchair. He didn't believe spine surgery was perfected enough in those days, and he thought it would be too risky. As for my parents, well, in those days, parents didn't really want to own up to their children's problems. Mine sent me to modeling school—they just thought scoliosis was something that would go away. As a result, I pretty much had to figure out what to do on my own.

By the time I was thirty-eight, I was in terrible pain all the time. After each pregnancy, I gained about sixty pounds, and having to carry my children around just seemed to throw me off. My curve was getting worse, but I still couldn't find a doctor who'd do the surgery—they all thought I was too old, and I suppose they were worried about malpractice, too. I got really discouraged. "I guess I waited too long," I'd say to my husband. "Nobody's going to operate on a grandma."

Finally, after a lot of probing, I found a new doctor who took x-rays of my spine. The curve was about 70 degrees, and he said he couldn't see that there was any reason in the world why I couldn't have surgery. I was elated. I was primed for it. And I made an appointment for the surgery. But so many people kept telling me I was nuts to go through with such a serious surgery, I eventually changed my mind and canceled it. I just figured I could live with the pain.

I couldn't. The pain got really bad—sort of a burning sensation in my back and a numbness in my legs. So I went back to the doctor, and he said he'd operate on me and put in a Harrington rod to straighten me out. I'd done a lot of research, though, and knew that sometimes a lumbar curve like mine can wind up looking unnaturally flat when a Harrington rod is inserted, and that it might tilt my body forward. So I decided to get a second opinion. What did I have to lose? The doctor told me it would be better for my particular curve to have two operations—an anterior and a posterior with Luque wires. So I decided to go *ahead with it, and in January I checked into the hospital. I had a lot of nightmares about the surgeries. I always imagined that I'd wake up a paraplegic or something. I just kept thinking, "I'm bad now, but am I going to be worse off afterward?"*

I can't say I had any real pain after the first surgery. I was so heavily sedated, I can't really remember. But to me, the hardest part of the two-stage procedure is the psychological part, knowing that after you've made it through the first one, you've got to get ready for a second one. I felt as if I was going to crumble, and I wouldn't wish that feeling on anyone. But there was a chaplain in the hospital who came to see me every day. He was marvelous! One of the most supportive men I think I've ever met. He was there just for me and made me feel as though everything was going to be wonderful. That was a big help, because my husband couldn't be there the entire time. It was nice to know that if you cried, you wouldn't have to cry alone.

Everything went fine with both surgeries, and, three weeks later, I got fitted for my brace and was allowed to go home. But the recuperation period was tough because I was home alone most of the time. I did hire a day-care person to come in to make the beds each day, and occasionally an R.N. stopped by to see how I was doing, but I mostly had to do everything myself. After the second week at home, in fact, I did all my own cooking and practically all of the cleaning.

I didn't have that much pain once I got home. Of course, the surgery is sort of like having a baby—you forget the pain very soon! I did feel a burning sensation where they did the fusion, but I just took a couple of extra-strength Tylenol and that took care of the problem. I think I'm a fast healer. I bounced back very quickly after surgery. After just three and a half months, I was doing all the lawn work and gardening—even trimming all the shrubbery with electric shears. And now, just five months after surgery, I'm in the process of stripping off all our wallpaper so that I can repaint the walls!

Now that my curve is about 35 degrees—half of what it used to be— I can wear dresses with a waistline and no one knows that I ever had scoliosis. I used to be so ashamed, having to wear dresses that were too big for me in order to hide my curve. The first time I went out to buy a dress after surgery was the most wonderful experience in the world—I didn't have to hide in the fitting room!

Today I think my overall appearance is great, but because they had to fuse the lower part of my spine, I don't think my gait is as natural as it used to be. When I walk slowly, like when you're walking up an aisle, I notice that I'm a little off-balance. I feel stiffer and can't move the way I did before. And even though the doctors told me this before surgery, it still bothers me. It's something you just have to get used to.

Every so often, someone will ask me whether or not they should have surgery. If a person has the choice to have the surgery done early in life, I'd say go for it!

FAMILY AND FRIENDS PROVIDE INVALUABLE SUPPORT

Laney M., seventeen, is one of many youngsters who were wise enough to go for surgery at an early age. But first, she tried everything she could to avoid it:

When I went for my yearly checkup at thirteen, my doctor didn't notice that I had a curvature. But a month later, my gymnastics coach pointed it out. I wasn't all that surprised, because when I used to do handsprings or walkovers, I'd get these sharp pains in my back. I kind of thought something might be wrong.

So we went to an orthopedist and found out that I had a 28-degree curve. I had to wear a Boston brace—which I named Oscar—for about a year. I never took it off, except for half an hour every day to take a shower. And I did lots of exercises, too, even while I was wearing it. After about six months, Oscar had reduced the size of my curve. But when I had x-rays taken at the end of the year, my curve was getting close to 40 degrees. By then, my shoulder jutted out toward the front about three inches, and I always had to stand in a certain way to try to look straight. The doctor said we'd have to start thinking about surgery.

Everybody told me it was up to me to decide, but I said, "It's not up to me, because there's nothing I personally can do about it." I just had to face it, because I didn't want my curve to get any worse. I didn't really know what the doctors were going to do to me, but the night before surgery, they showed me a film that explained more about it. I started getting worried, but both my parents were there, and a bunch of friends called to say good luck, so it wasn't that bad. If my parents hadn't been there, it would have been bad, I think, because it can be scary and it helps to have someone to talk to.

I wasn't scared the morning of the surgery, except when they were taking me down to the operating room and at one point they told my parents they couldn't walk with me any farther. Then I started crying, but I really don't know what I was afraid of. I don't like shots—I'm a big baby when it comes to stuff like that. I think I got scared because I didn't know what was going to happen. So I just kept asking the doctors, "You're not going to hurt me, are you?" They all said no, they wouldn't hurt me. And then someone gave me a shot to put me to sleep, and I don't remember a thing until I got to my regular hospital room.

The doctors had told me that I'd hurt afterward, and they were right. After surgery [which involved a Harrington rod affixed with wires], I was in a lot of pain—like a throbbing from below my butt up to my neck. But they do give you medicine and that makes you feel better.

It took quite a while to get my strength back. For five or six days after surgery, I just ate ice chips and was real weak. I was starving, but once I got my food, I didn't feel like eating it. My stomach was upset, and I couldn't go to the bathroom. So when they wheeled me down to get the plaster mold fitted for my brace, my legs were shaking and I could hardly stand up. It was really hard, but it helped that my dad was there with me.

Once I got home, I would get really tired. But I stayed in bed hardly at all. I was moving around the house, doing my walking exercises a lot. I didn't feel like doing my homework, but I had a homebound tutor who helped me. I also ate a lot. Because I'd lost about fifteen pounds after surgery, my mom fed me steak for breakfast, lunch, and dinner—which sounds good, but you do get sick of it after a while.

Although the doctor said I could go back to school two weeks after surgery, I waited six weeks so I could start a new term. All the kids were *really nice when I got back, and they hardly noticed my brace because it's so form-fitting. Even the really popular kids, the ones you don't think know who you are, said, "Hey, Laney, we're glad you're back at school." And the only class I had trouble catching up on was Spanish, but that's because everything you learn in a foreign language builds on everything else.*

The saddest thing to me is that I had to give up gymnastics. I never did think I was going to be all that great, but I just liked the sport. We went to meets three nights a week, out of town, and I miss seeing all those people. But now I'm taking up tennis—I've played three times since surgery—and I'm pretty good at it.

Even though I was in a lot of pain after surgery—sometimes I thought I was going to die—I can hardly remember any of it now. My brace came off after only four months, I got an inch and a half taller, I've finally got a waistline, and now I'm straight. And in another couple of weeks, after the doctor has checked out my x-rays, I'm looking forward to getting his permission to go water-skiing!

Laney's mother, Catherine, looks forward to that day as well. For her, it will mark the end of the family's bout with scoliosis, an experience that seemed to last "forever." Here, she shares some thoughts about what it's like to be the parent of a youngster who's going to have scoliosis surgery:

We felt relieved when we learned that Laney could have surgery. We'd been living with the brace for such a long time, and it was uncomfortable, cumbersome, and hot for Laney. As a mother, it had hurt me to watch her wearing the Boston brace, and we'd had such problems trying to find her clothes that would fit—the brace made her waist three sizes bigger, but her hips were so tiny, everything would just fall to the floor. She accepted it pretty well—we had our "Oscar designer clothes" and all—but it was hard for her. It seemed like she'd been in that brace forever, and we were glad that something else could be done for her.

Her curve was just going wild. Over the summer, it increased 20 more degrees in her lower back, and she was getting a bad inward slope in the middle of her back. That scared me, because it increased even though she swam every day and was wearing a brace. I could tell how bad it was getting—when she'd dive in the swimming pool, her back would go crooked. And I knew if we didn't do something, it would only get worse.

When we knew she was going to have surgery, we got on the ball right away to get things done, like having Laney donate her own blood for the surgery. But where we live, you can't donate blood if you're underage, so we had a lot of problems—it was almost as if it took an act of Congress. It can be done, though. We got permission from our pediatrician and from the orthopedic surgeon, and had to go through the state Red Cross to get approval. Then we had to drive sixty miles every week to give the blood.

My husband and I worked it out so that one of us was with Laney all the time she was in the hospital. I was able to stay near her overnight, and in the morning, when I went back to the hotel to shower, my husband would come over and stay with her. I think it helped her a lot. When she had gas pains, I was there to rub her stomach and walk her up and down the halls with the IV still attached to her arm; when she had to have the plaster mold put on, her daddy went with her. That seemed to make her feel better.

Several things happened that made us all feel better. First, we brought our hometown orthopedic surgeon to the hospital so he could watch the surgery. We wanted to make sure he'd know what to do if we had problems once we got home. Second, everything was out in the open—everything that was told to my husband and me was told to Laney, and I think that's the way it should be. We never had any secrets, and I think that's why she handled it as well as she did. Third, our surgeon could bring himself down to the eye level of the patient. He commands respect, but he can communicate with a child. I liked that and felt it was important to Laney.

I know that some parents are afraid to bring their kids to the doctor. But the one thing I've learned through this is that you must take a child—or an adult, for that matter—to the doctor when she's healthy. That way you'll have records that you can refer to so you know what's wrong. If you wait until there's something wrong, it may be too late.

SURGERIES STRAIGHTENED THE SPINE AND STRENGTHENED THE CHARACTER

Like many of the surgical patients I interviewed, I put off having surgery until I was an adult. I finally made the decision at the age of twenty, nearly five years after I had first sensed something was wrong with my back. That's unfortunate, because at the age of fifteen, my curve was probably only 20 degrees and could have been treated nonoperatively. By the time I met a spine specialist, my spine had twisted around to 43 degrees. I felt surgery was my only alternative.

My deformity was not obvious to the casual observer. I did not have the rib hump that is often associated with severe scoliosis, but my torso did seem to be twisting to the left, the result of a mild rotation of the vertebrae. And though my right shoulder was nearly an inch higher than my left, as was my hip, by deliberately leaning in the opposite direction, I could compensate for the asymmetry and make my body appear to be nearly level. Compensating for my crookedness, however, was a full-time, tiresome job; standing straight and level did not come naturally to me.

Curves like mine, in the 40- to 60-degree range, are not life-threatening. In most cases, they don't interfere with the heart or lungs, and rarely do they cause pain. Indeed, many adults have curves of this magnitude, but they elect to do nothing about them. They can live with the fact that their bodies are slightly off-kilter. But there is a chance that curves can get worse during adulthood. That such a possibility existed was what made me decide to go ahead with surgery.

It was not an easy decision to make. I had just enrolled as a freshman at the University of Minnesota and was working two part-time jobs as a legal secretary in order to finance my plans to one day become an English teacher. I'd also just met a fellow whom I thought would be the man of my dreams. Surgery threatened to ruin all of that. It would mean dropping out of school and work for a while: in those days, the standard recuperation period was at least a month. And, since patients at that time typically wore a plaster body cast for many months, I knew I'd be putting my newfound relationship in jeopardy. For weeks I was in agony: should I have the surgery and get "fixed," or should I gamble that my curve would stay right where it was?

On the strength of five years of painful memories and the sneaking suspicion that with my luck, the curve would worsen, I decided to go through with it. On a January evening, I checked into Fairview–St. Mary's Hospital at five-feet-two, and by ten o'clock the next morning, thanks to Dr. David Bradford's expert bone-carpentry skills and the insertion of a Harrington rod, I was five-feet-four, though quite unconscious of my newly heightened stature.

When I finally awoke many hours later, one thought drifted through my mind: "I'm now two inches taller than I was a few hours ago." But as the anesthesia wore off and my body became more attuned to the realities of major surgery, all I could think of was pain. I felt as if someone were standing on my torso. I called for more pain medication and got it, then drifted back to sleep.

A few days later, when I started to feel a bit more alert, two nurses stood at my bedside and announced, "It's time for your log rolls." I didn't know what they were talking about, until one of them pulled up the sheet beneath me and used it like a lever to roll me to the other side, where the other nurse stood ready to catch me.

"Don't do that!" I screamed. "I'm not ready to move yet! You're going to break my rod!" They assured me that log rolls were good for me. As for the Harrington rod hooked to my spine, they said it wouldn't break. "It's made of stainless steel," they said.

They were right. The rod didn't break, and by week's end, I came to look forward to seeing their cheery faces as they clutched at my sheet and shouted, "Alley-oop!" I would have gladly gone along with being rolled indefinitely if it had meant I could escape the next traumatic experience that awaited me. I was wheeled down to the cast room, where four orthopedic residents were preparing to slather my body with the sticky, smelly goop that would harden and become my body cast.

"What kind of body do you want?" they asked. "Voluptuous? Streamlined? If you've got the time, we've got the plaster." Jokesters, all of them. But their playful banter helped allay my fears as they removed my surgical gown, pulled a long body stocking over my head, and positioned it, like an elongated tube top, over two-thirds of my shivering body. Unable to see what they were about to do—the top of the stocking covered my face to protect it from clouds of plaster dust—I prayed for time to pass quickly. Within minutes, they were patting and pulling long strips of plaster-soaked gauze around my neck and across my breasts, waist, and hips.

"More on the left!" one of them shouted. "Smooth down the buttocks," said another. "Aren't you finished yet?" I mumbled beneath my mask.

Twenty minutes later, the plaster had dried. I lay there on the table, my face finally exposed to the light, feeling like a mummy—cold, clammy, encased. But before I had a chance to whine about it, one of the residents was coming toward me with what looked like a little buzz saw.

"What are you going to do with that?" I gasped.

"Trim your hair, dummy," he said with a giggle. "Seriously, I'm just going to trim your cast. You want to look good in this, don't you?" He zipped off the excess plaster from around my neck, shoulders, and buttocks, then cut out a large oval from the plaster that surrounded my stomach.

"This will help you breathe easily," he said. "You'll be glad it's there after you eat. When your stomach expands, it'll have somewhere to go." When he finished with his nips and tucks, the group hoisted me back on the cart and returned me to my room.

I wasn't allowed to get out of bed yet, so I couldn't see what the cast looked like, but I was dying to know. Was it really as big as it felt? How was I going to conceal it? I was certain I looked hideous, but I wouldn't know for sure for another week.

"It's time to get out of bed and take your first walk," said my nurse about two weeks after the surgery. The news stunned me. I felt no more prepared to walk than I did to play football! But despite my protests, I soon found myself on the edge of the bed, my feet dangling toward the floor.

"Up you go!" said my nurse. "C'mon. You can do it!"

What a bizarre feeling to stand again! My knees were wobbling and I felt as if my body would buckle under the weight of the twelve-pound cast. Slowly I took one step, then another. Two steps later, I was ready to sit down. But before I did, I managed to gather enough strength to walk to a mirror. I had to see what I looked like!

"Hideous!" I thought as I stroked the boxy mold that hid my otherwise tiny figure. "I look like a freak!"

No one could comfort me. Not the nurses, not Dr. Bradford, least of all my friends. They all said I looked fine ("for somebody who's just had spine surgery"), but I knew they were lying. I looked like a mummy and sure as hell felt like one. I pleaded with Dr. Bradford to remove it, trying to convince him that I'd be really careful if I didn't have to wear one. But he was unfazed by my arguments. "It's there to protect you," he reminded me. "You never know what might happen."

I didn't think I'd be able to stand it. And it was going to be like this for the next nine months! I was angry, hurt, and depressed. But worse, I was worried. What would my new boyfriend do or say when he saw me like this?

I got my answer three weeks later when he came to pick me up for our first date since the surgery. We were going to a party at the home of one of his friends, people I'd never met. That made me nervous, but not as much as seeing my date did. After all, he'd probably never seen a walking, talking mummy before!

To say that he looked surprised when he saw me would be an understatement. When I opened the door, he took one look at me and said, "Oh God, I didn't know it was going to look like that!" I tried to appear cheerful and even offered to let him sign my cast. "Maybe later," he said glumly as he led me to his car. We rode in silence. His eyes were glued to the road, mine on the ceiling of the car. That was the only position I could sit in where the cast didn't pinch into my chin.

When we arrived at the party, I felt as if everyone was staring at me. Indeed, they probably were, since none of them had ever seen a person in a body cast. "Doesn't it hurt?" "Aren't you hot?" "Do you really have to wear that thing for nine whole months?" Everyone had a question, and I got pretty sick of it, if you want to know the truth. So after about a half-hour of being grilled with queries, I fled to the bathroom and had a good cry. Finally I composed myself, yanked my turtleneck up over the neck piece one more time, and made my way down the basement stairs that led to the party room below.

Suddenly my ankle gave out on the second step and I fell back, sliding jerkily down the stairs on my back like a turtle skidding down a bumpy hill. The back of my head and my buttocks ached from hitting against the plaster as I made my descent. But nothing was hurt more than my pride.

They all flocked around me. "Are you all right?" "Are you hurt?" "Maybe somebody should call an ambulance!" Actually, that didn't strike me as such a bad idea—I wasn't seriously hurt but I sure wanted to make a fast getaway!

My date wasn't much help. In fact, I think he was more embarrassed than I was. But at least he was quick on his feet; he had me in the car within minutes, and we were on our way back to my apartment. We didn't speak, aware that this was probably our last date. But the twenty-minute ride gave me time to come to two important, startling realizations. Any guy who couldn't see through plaster to find the person underneath just wasn't the guy for me. And now I knew that my ugly, cumbersome shell was there for a reason after all. It probably saved me from breaking my neck, my rod, or my back!

By the next week, I had returned to school and my jobs. No, it wasn't easy schlepping around campus with this heavy shell surrounding my body, or craning my neck over the bulky mold in order to see what I was typing at work. I also disliked having to take sponge baths, and shampooing my hair meant getting into the bathtub on all fours with a plastic sheet wrapped around me to protect the plaster. The smell of sweaty plaster in the summer was enough to make me retch; even dumping spoonfuls of Chanel N°5 bathpowder down my back couldn't mask the odor! I hated the way I looked—I felt compelled to cover myself with turtlenecks and maternity tops, which only made me look worse, and pregnant. And sometimes I thought I'd go mad because of the itching. My solution to this problem was to stretch out a wire hanger and try to slip it underneath my cast, but it usually ended up getting caught on the body stocking, whereupon I'd be forced to ask a neighbor to help me pull it out! But despite all these aggravations, time passed quickly, and before I knew it, I was back in Dr. Bradford's office. The day of the unveiling had finally arrived.

No sound has ever been lovelier to me than that of the small buzz saw he used to remove my cast. In minutes, it was split open and the dusty, frayed shell, now in halves, fell to the floor. Quickly I ran my hands along my back. It felt good. It felt straight. But would it bend?

Slowly I leaned over from the waist, my hands dangling toward the floor. No pain, just a little stiffness from being held imprisoned all those months. Next, with my hands on my hips, I twisted at the waist, then arched my back. No problem! By now, I couldn't even remember where Dr. Bradford had placed the rod along my spine. I knew only that I now had terrific posture! At that moment, it mattered little that a four-hour operation, a metal rod, and a plaster torture chamber had made it possible.

When I returned home that afternoon, I ripped off my turtleneck, vowed to burn it and every other piece of "cast clothing" I owned, and slid into a steamy bubble bath, where I giddily watched every square inch of my skin shrivel up like a prune. That first bath could well be entered in the *Guinness Book of World Records* as the longest time any human has ever spent lounging in a tub! Then I spent several hours prancing nude around my living room, taking breaks every five minutes or so to admire my newly straightened body in the mirror. What a delightful time I had trying on all the clothes I hadn't worn for nearly a year and dreaming about all the new, slinky outfits I would buy that would adorn my lovely new body! To be sure, that day ranks among the top ten of my life.

Over the course of the next seven years, I finished my course work at the university, completed my apprenticeship as a student teacher, and started teaching English at a high school in a suburb of Minneapolis. That was a year of triumph for me because it marked the first year of what I thought would be a lifetime career. But it was also a year of anguish: the Harrington rod inside me broke, and once again I was faced with having to have surgery.

I firmly believe I know exactly when it happened, though Dr. Bradford contends that the rod probably began to wear out over a period of months, that it would be unlikely to snap suddenly, or that a person would actually feel it break. Both of us, however, agree on why it happened: A small portion of the bone graft had failed to fuse years before (in an area of my spine that was not easily seen on x-ray), and this caused the rod to become dislodged and more susceptible to stress, the way a hairpin, if continually twisted, will eventually weaken and break.

One breezy summer evening, I was sitting in an overstuffed chair in my apartment, correcting huge piles of research papers I had assigned my students as their final project of the year. Suddenly I heard a crash in the next room and reeled around in my chair, certain that a burglar had climbed in through the bedroom window. Midway through my turn, I felt a hot pain shoot up my spine, not unlike the painful tingling sensation you feel when you turn your neck too quickly. Slightly dazed, I got up from my chair, tiptoed toward the bedroom, and saw that the wind had blown my tiny wind chime against the wall and shattered it. I began cleaning up the mess, but when I bent over to pick up the shards of glass, I felt that tingling sensation again.

When I awoke the next morning, my entire upper body felt stiff and my head throbbed. And in the days that followed, although the stiffness disappeared, the headache became my constant companion. Rest did not relieve the pain. Great quantities of aspirin had no effect. Nothing took the pain away.

Because it was my head, not my back, that hurt, it didn't occur to me at first that something might be wrong with my spine. In fact, when I finally made an appointment with a general practitioner, I never even mentioned that I'd had spine surgery. All I talked about was the throbbing in my head.

Believing that my problem was tension, the doctor wrote out a prescription for Valium, a muscle relaxant. Dutifully, I took one every four hours, but the drug didn't rid me of my headache; it only made me feel groggy and depressed.

After weeks of wooziness, I decided that my problem was not tension. God knows, popping all that Valium made my body feel like rubber most of the time! So I finally made an appointment with Dr. Bradford. Perhaps all this pain did have something to do with my back.

I'll never forget that day. Dr. Bradford sent me to the lab for x-rays and when I returned to his office, I slipped on a flimsy paper gown while he quickly examined my body and listened to my tale of the twenty-four-hour-a-day headaches. My body checked out fine, he said, and so I stood behind a privacy screen and began getting dressed. In the meantime, a nurse delivered the x-rays, and Dr. Bradford put them up on the light board. just as I zipped up my slacks, I heard him say, "Hmmm, your rod's broken."

I peeked around the screen and looked at the x-ray. Seemingly floating amid the cloudy-looking vertebrae was a rod—half of it secured in place against the spine, the other half jutting out at an angle where the break had occurred. "Surely that couldn't be *my* x-ray," I thought. "That wasn't *my* rod, was it?"

Dr. Bradford gently assured me that the x-ray and the rod indeed belonged to me.

"I'm sorry this happened," he said, pointing to the two pieces that were once a single shaft of metal. "It's happened because you've got a pseudoarthrosis—one part of your fusion didn't take." I don't recall hearing him explain that when pseudoarthrosis occurs, part of your spine buckles out and puts pressure on the rod, which in turn causes it to break. I only remember these words: "We're going to have to go back in and repair the fusion and put in a new rod."

Today, if an adult patient experiences pseudoarthrosis or has another type of condition that requires a revision of a fusion, the surgeon may recommend that he or she wear a spinal stimulator after surgery for several hours a day for a period of three to five months. According to Dr. Frank Rand of Boston Children's Hospital, who notes that these electromagnetic devices have been approved by FDA, and that, "although we're not quite sure why they work, spinal stimulators can improve a patient's fusion rate. We don't typically recommend its use for a first surgery, but if I were doing a revision of a fusion, or any type of fusion in the pelvic area, I would definitely think about using it. Patients who think they might benefit from a stimulator should consult with their orthopedists."

Back to my own experience. Quite frankly, I didn't care about the surgery or the rod. What mattered to me was the fact that, once again, I'd be enveloped in a plaster cast. Nine more months of looking like a cocoon!

I can't say I enjoyed this second ordeal, yet I have to admit I was pleasantly surprised at the way things turned out. In the seven years since I'd had my first surgery, doctors had changed their thinking about how postsurgical patients should be treated, so this time, instead of lying on my back in my body cast for weeks after surgery, I was up and walking after about three days. I was out of the hospital seven days later and returned to teaching within two weeks, this time in a much thinner cast that just barely covered my collarbone and stopped at the middle of my hips.

Psychologically, I was a much stronger patient the second time around. During the seven months that I wore the cast, I didn't try to conceal myself in turtlenecks or maternity tops, and in fact, I made a conscious effort to dress just like anyone else, even if portions of the cast did peek through my clothes. I even got used to being teased by my students—they loved to tell me "knock-knock" jokes while rapping on my cast and shrieking, "Who's there?"

Of course, I wouldn't want to go through surgery again. Twice is enough for anybody! But what I gained from the experience of having two spine surgeries and wearing body casts for a total of sixteen months of my life has more than offset any of the fear, anguish, and pain I had to endure as the result of having had scoliosis. I'm not referring here to the physical benefits of surgery—the fact that I'm still two inches taller, have great posture, two evenly balanced shoulders, a clearly defined waist, and no longer have to struggle with clothes that don't seem to fit. What is important to me is the psychological and emotional strength I garnered along the way.

In ways that may be difficult for someone who hasn't had surgery to understand, scoliosis *can* strengthen your character. Who can fear a deadline or a test, a meeting or a confrontation, after one experiences and overcomes the fear of having a surgeon work so close to the spinal cord? Who can be plagued by self-consciousness in everyday situations after one has sported a brace—or a heavy plaster cast—all summer long? And who can be impatient with the little aggravations of daily existence after one has waited months to be released from a protective shell?

If you have never had great respect for the human body and your health, or taken your share of responsibility for these marvelous gifts of life, you're a lot like I was before I finally had to come to grips with the fact that I'd have to have surgery. But once you have taken steps to correct your scoliosis—by making an appointment with a specialist, being fitted for a brace, or going through with surgery if you need it—you will be that much closer to taking control of your life—a long, happy, productive life that is the result of stopping scoliosis in time.

6

Adult Scoliosis

t has been estimated that as many as two to four million adults in the United States have scoliosis. While the majority of these are people with curves under 30 degrees that are not progressing and never need treatment, it is important to know that they did not suddenly develop the disorder later in life. With the exception of people who develop degenerative scoliosis, most adults who now have scoliosis probably have idiopathic scoliosis and developed their curves in adolescence.

This chapter addresses adult scoliosis, which is a condition in which rotation of the spinal vertebrae leads to curvature of the spine in a person who has finished growing (growth is usually completed between the ages of eighteen and twenty-one years). In order to be classified as scoliosis, the curve must exceed 10 degrees. Curves can occur in the thoracic spine or the lumbar spine. Occasionally, curves involve areas of the spine that lie in between. The cervical spine is rarely involved.

To find out more about this important topic, I consulted with Dennis Crandall, M.D., an orthopedic spine surgeon who is medical director of the Sonoran Spine Center in Phoenix, Arizona, and attending surgeon for the Scoliosis Clinic at Children's Rehabilitative Services in Phoenix. Not long ago, he wrote an extensive article on the subject for *Backtalk,* the newsletter of The Scoliosis Association. The information that follows is based on that article.

Q: *Are there different types of adult scoliosis?*

A: When curvature of the spine starts in adolescence in an otherwise healthy person, it is most commonly diagnosed as idiopathic scoliosis. *Idiopathic* refers to the fact that the curve is not associated with other known problems, such as cerebral palsy, spina bifida, neurofibromatosis, or a number of other conditions. After age eighteen, the idiopathic scoliosis is termed *adult idiopathic scoliosis.* It is the same curve present during the teen years, but the adult spine does not behave in the same way as the teenage spine. As a person with scoliosis ages, the spine develops premature aging changes such as bone spurs, degenerative discs, and thickened spinal ligaments. This leads to a condition known as *adult idiopathic scoliosis with degenerative changes.* These degenerative changes, superimposed on a curve that is already present, can sometimes cause back pain, leg pain, spinal imbalance, and progression or worsening of the curve. For adult curves greater than 50 degrees, our natural history studies suggest that they have a high likelihood of progressing about 1 degree per year. For curves in the lumbar spine or lower back, there is a high chance of progression if the curve is greater than about 40 degrees.

Q: *What is degenerative scoliosis?*

A: Degenerative scoliosis is connected to age-related changes in the spine. As arthritis begins to affect the spine, the intervertebral discs lose their water content and consequently their ability to serve as "shock absorbers." The facet joints in the back of the spine begin to wear out and lose their ability to maintain normal spinal alignment. The vertebrae begin to slip or move abnormally. This may lead to spinal instability, nerve compression, and pain. As both the discs and the facet joints lose their ability to maintain normal spinal motion, the spine can settle asymmetrically, leading to scoliosis. If a person's lumbar spine was straight as an adult but develops a curve later in life (usually after the age of sixty), it is termed *de novo scoliosis,* referring to spontaneous development of scoliosis due to degeneration of the joints and discs in the spine. This can occur at younger ages in people who have undergone the type of spine surgery known as *laminectomy,* in which portions of the vertebral bone is removed to decompress pinched nerves. However, it never occurs without significant arthritis.

Q: *What are the signs and symptoms of adult scoliosis?*
A: The most common sign of adult scoliosis is a prominence in the ribs on one side of the thoracic spine. In the lumbar spine, there is sometimes a prominence on one side, though often there is not. The prominence, or rib hump, is most apparent when the person bends forward. Sometimes there is an asymmetry in the waist, with one side being indented more than the other. Clothes begin to fit differently than they used to.

If the scoliosis is severe and unstable, spinal imbalance is common. You may lean to one side or forward when you try to stand straight upright; you may feel like you are tipping to one side or have a constant sense that you are falling forward. Most people with adult scoliosis notice that they are not as tall as they used to be.

Most young adults with scoliosis do not have significant back pain. The curve usually does not hurt unless or until it becomes degenerative. Sometime in life, however, because arthritis is age related and develops prematurely in people with scoliosis, back pain may develop. When it occurs, the pain is worse when a person is upright and active, and better when he or she is resting. Spinal instability occurs when the disc and facet joints are so worn out that they can no longer maintain normal spinal alignment. Pain comes from the arthritic joints as well as from

the adjacent nerves, which are pinched and stretched as a
result.

Pain in the buttocks can occur due to referred pain from the
arthritic spine. It can also be a manifestation of a more significant problem with nerve compression. Spinal nerve roots become pinched when arthritic bone spurs form around them and
block their exit route from the spinal column. This condition is
called *spinal stenosis*. In addition to buttock pain, other symptoms—such as leg pain, numbness, tingling, and weakness—
are common. If you develop any of these symptoms, you should
seek a physician's advice without delay.

If spinal stenosis or nerve compression in the back is severe
enough, control of bowel and bladder function will be lost.
Thankfully, this is rare, but when it happens, it signals a surgical emergency. If the pressure on the nerves is not relieved
quickly, bladder and bowel control may never be regained.

Q: *What are some of the challenges adults with scoliosis face?*
A: As the spine ages, it becomes stiffer. Flexibility is greatest in
   the teen years and usually declines starting in a person's forties
   or fifties. In adults with scoliosis, spinal stiffness can become
   severe as bone spurs form and prohibit motion. In some cases,
   the bone-spur formation is so severe that all motion is lost at
   one or more levels in the spine.

   We all achieve our maximum bone density between the ages
   of thirty and thirty-five. After age thirty-five to forty, there is a
   slow decline in the amount of bone present in the spine. After
   age sixty, and particularly after menopause in women, the loss
   of bone becomes visible on x-rays. This is osteoporosis. If the
   bone loss becomes severe, spontaneous fractures can occur in
   the spine. These fractures can lead to scoliosis or kyphosis.

   As we age, our general health can become more of a problem. Chronic diseases such as high blood pressure, diabetes,
   and heart disease are prevalent among American seniors. If
   scoliosis becomes a problem for an adult, particularly an older

adult, other health issues must be taken into account when treatment options are considered.

Q: *Are there conservative treatments available for adults with scoliosis?*
A: Nearly all people with adult scoliosis respond to conservative treatment and can lead a normal, functional life. If pain is present, it is usually short-term and manageable. Treatment for adult scoliosis should almost always begin with a noninvasive approach. I say, "Try the easy things first."

Nonsteroidal anti-inflammatory drugs (NSAIDs) have long been the cornerstone of medical therapy for arthritic and inflammatory conditions. These medications can quiet the pain and relieve stiffness caused by degenerating discs and joints.

Physical therapy is an excellent way to improve function, flexibility, and endurance, and to decrease pain. Usually, a therapist will work toward reducing your symptoms and will recommend an active home exercise program to maintain the improvement. Working out in a supervised environment with the help of a physical therapist is the best way to achieve this. On average, therapy sessions are scheduled for two to three times per week for four to eight weeks.

It is very important that adults with scoliosis get into the habit of doing a *daily* exercise routine. This will improve the strength of the trunk muscles and take some of the stress off the spine. Often, when pain occurs, it is because the individual is not doing his or her exercises.

For some people with degenerative scoliosis, a back brace can be helpful in providing relief from back pain. A word of caution is in order, however: The brace should not be used without faithful compliance with an active exercise program. Wearing a brace without exercise tends to lead to a weaker spine that becomes dependent on the brace. Exercising daily and wearing the brace occasionally, when needed, lead to the best results where bracing is concerned.

Medical management of osteoporosis and general health is

important for maintaining an active lifestyle into older adult-hood, especially for people with scoliosis. Solving small prob-lems before they become big ones has always been good advice.

Q: *When might surgery be considered?*

A: Few people with adult scoliosis ultimately require surgery. When it does become necessary, however, the goals of surgery are to stop the progression of the curve(s), stabilize the spine, establish correct spinal balance, decrease back and leg pain, and increase function, with as little surgery and as few compli-cations as possible. People who require surgery to straighten, stabilize, and fuse their spinal curvature are those who have:

1. A curvature that is increasing over time (it will continue to get worse);
2. An unstable spine that hurts despite conservative care;
3. Nerve compression that is causing pain, numbness, or weakness;
4. A spinal imbalance that is painful or progressive; and/or
5. A large curve that will progress. (In such cases, it's better to have surgery earlier, while the person's health is good and before osteoporosis starts or worsens.)

Q: *What are some of the surgical options?*

A: If the main problem is leg pain resulting from disc herniation, this can usually be taken care of with a small procedure to re-move the disc fragment and decompress the nerve. A larger procedure to correct the scoliosis and fuse the spine is not necessary.

   Sometimes leg pain is caused by bone spurs that are com-pressing the spinal nerves. This is spinal stenosis. If stenosis is the problem, the solution usually requires removal of offending bone spurs to relieve pain. If enough bone is surgically removed to decompress the pinched nerves (laminectomy), the spine is often rendered unstable in the process. Back pain may increase, leg pain may return, and the spinal curvature will get bigger if the spine is not fused at the same time. In such cases, correction of the curve and fusion with bone graft and instrumentation are required to stabilize the spine and prevent what would be a certain need for future surgery.

If back pain, progressive deformity, and/or spinal imbalance are primary factors, the curve should be straightened and fused. Unfortunately, the amount of correction obtained with surgery in adults is generally less than that seen in children and adolescents because the spine becomes increasingly stiff in adulthood.

Q: *What surgical techniques are used to correct adult scoliosis?*
A: Once the decision to have surgery has been made, an operative plan is formulated. Patients are routinely asked to donate blood before surgery to be stored and used during their surgery. The spinal cord is usually monitored throughout the surgery to make sure there is no compromise to spinal cord function.

Surgery to correct adult scoliosis is the most challenging surgery done in orthopedics and is likely among the most complex and demanding surgeries of any kind performed today. This type of surgery requires at least one assisting surgeon and, often, a surgical team, and can take from four to fourteen hours to accomplish.

If the spine must be fused anteriorly, or from the front, a thoracic or general surgeon will be included in the surgical team to safely mobilize the great blood vessels off the spine where the spine surgeon will work. The incision may be made through the side of the chest, through the side of the abdomen, or through the front of the abdomen, depending on what is needed at the time of surgery The purpose of anterior surgery is to remove the discs and fill the space with bone graft. This serves to improve the correction that can be achieved and improve the reliability of the fusion. Sometimes the spine is "instrumented" from the front, meaning that screws are placed into the vertebrae and attached to a rod that will correct the

deformity and stabilize the spine. More recently, the thoracoscope has been used in spine surgery. We can now remove discs
from the thoracic spine and insert bone graft without making a
large incision. All of the work is done through a few one-inch
incisions on the side of the chest.

Most of the correction of adult scoliosis is done posteriorly,
or from the back of the spine. If nerves are compressed by bone
spurs or a herniated disc, the offending spurs or discs can be
removed to allow more room for the nerves. The spine is then
"instrumented" by the placement of hooks or screws that attach
to the vertebrae. These hooks and screws are then attached to
rods that span the curve. The instrumentation is then dis-
tracted, compressed, or rotated in order to correct the spinal
curvature. Without instrumentation, the curve cannot be
corrected.

Bone graft is always used in scoliosis surgery. The spine must
be fused in its new corrected and straightened position. The
graft most commonly comes from the patient's own pelvis.
Sometimes bone-bank bone is used. This is usually resorted to
if there is not sufficient bone available from the patient.

Q: *What sort of results can people with adult scoliosis expect from
surgery?*

A: Adults who undergo major spine surgery to correct scoliosis
generally do well. Most experience relief of pain. Fusion is usually successful, and the correction is maintained long-term in
80 to 95 percent of people who undergo correction of mild to
moderate scoliosis, with or without nerve root decompression.

As with any type of surgery, however, there can be complications. Potential complications of scoliosis surgery include failure of the spine to fuse solidly, failure of the spine hardware
(experienced by some 5 percent of patients), infection (2 to 5
percent), nerve injury (somewhat more than 1 percent), medical complications, and others. People who are at greatest risk
for complications are those who smoke, those who take

steroids, and those who have severe osteoporosis or are poorly nourished.

We recently presented to the Scoliosis Research Society and the North American Spine Society the results of three different studies of adult patients with stiff degenerative scoliosis. All required fusion with instrumentation of the lumbar spine to the sacrum. Several had severe spinal imbalance. A full two years after their surgery, all patients reported significant improvement in their pain. Their need for narcotic pain medication decreased from 73 percent of patients before surgery to 9 percent after surgery. The techniques used were considered successful and promising.

Q: *Any thoughts about the future of spine surgery?*

A: On the horizon, there are several new technologies that are very exciting and will likely change the way we currently address spinal deformity. One of the most revolutionary concepts is the use of a substance known as *bone morphogenic protein (BMP)* to assist the spine in achieving a solid fusion. Look for BMP to be available to surgeons on a limited basis (outside of research programs) very soon.

Look for the spine surgery of the future to be safer, with fewer complications and better results than anything we now do. Spine surgery has made light-years of progress in just the past fifteen years. The future looks just as bright, if not brighter.

7

Scoliosis on the World Wide Web

If you have access to a computer, you've got a world of information about scoliosis right at your fingertips. What's out there on the Net? To find out, I consulted with Linda Racine of El Granada, California. She's a business executive—and a scoliosis patient—who keeps a watchful eye on hundreds of Internet sites dealing with scoliosis. As she told me, "You can find anything from snake oil to medical doctor opinions via the Internet. It's important, however, to understand that since the Internet is essentially unregulated, there are a lot of scams and an immense amount of misinformation along with medically proven treatments and helpful information. The trick is to be skeptical and apply one's common sense when viewing Internet sites."

There is no way to include all Internet sites dealing with scoliosis in this chapter, as new sites are created almost daily. So I asked Linda to categorize sites and give readers some samples of the better sites in each category:

Links to Scoliosis Sites

There are quite a number of Internet search engines available (for example, Yahoo.com, Search.com, Lycos.com, Iwon.com, and so on). A current search on the word *scoliosis,* using any of these search sites, will produce links to 25,000 Internet pages. One scoliosis site, Scoliosis World (www.scoliosis-world.com), is doing a great job of tracking scoliosis sites.

GENERAL SCOLIOSIS INFORMATION

This is the largest category of Internet sites that we viewed. There are hundreds of sites that describe what scoliosis is and what treatments are available. Many of these sites have excellent graphics that will help a person with scoliosis to understand his or her condition. Following are examples of sites in this category.

National Institute of Arthritis and Musculoskeletal and Skin Diseases
www.nih.gov/niams/healthinfo/scochild.htm
This site contains very easy-to-read and understandable information on scoliosis. Of particular value is a list of questions you might ask a potential surgeon.

Orthospine
www.orthospine.com/med_topics.htm
This is the website of a New York spine medical practice (many spine groups have their own websites). This site includes detailed sections on flat-back syndrome, herniated discs, spinal stenosis, low back pain, endoscopic surgery, kyphosis, spondylolisthesis, and spine aging. The use of clear graphics and x-rays make this site easy to navigate and comprehend.

Scoliosis Research Society (SRS)
www.srs.org/htm/library/review/review00.htm
The Library section of the SRS site has the best basic information on scoliosis and kyphosis. There are drawings, photos, and x-rays on every page,
which helps the reader understand what is often too technical for the
layperson.

Spine-Health
www.spine-health.com
This is an excellent site for general spine information. Of special interest
are animations that show back conditions and surgical treatments. The site
also contains a discussion forum that is moderated by medical professionals.

SpineUniverse
www.spineuniverse.com
This site provides articles on just about every type of traditional and alternative treatment available. Although it doesn't have basic information
such as you will find on the SRS or Orthospine sites, SpineUniverse has
an immense amount of information for both the medical and patient com-
munities. We were able to find articles on just about anything and everything to do with the spine. The articles are well written and informative.
Of particular interest to some will be the videos of many spine surgery
techniques.

BRACES AND BRACING

There are relatively few sites dealing with bracing, but the following is
worth checking out:

Journal of Prosthetics and Orthotics (JPO)
www.oandp.org/jpo/index.htm
This is the address for a listing of JPO articles on scoliosis. This site has
links to ten years worth of published articles. Of particular interest are ar-

ticles such as "Biomechanical Comparison of the Milwaukee Brace (CTLSO) and the TLSO for Treatment of Idiopathic Scoliosis." You can access this article at www.oandp.org/jpo/library/1966_04_115.asp.

CHAT

There are an abundance of sites that facilitate discussions about scoliosis. You can select the format of your choice: bulletin boards (where messages are viewable at your leisure); live chats (where you must be present at a specific time to participate); or e-mail lists (which send messages to everyone subscribed to the list). Following are some of the more popular sites.

Scoliosis Mailing List
www.ai.mit.edu/extra/scoliosis//scoliosis.html
This is actually six e-mail lists. Because many people have subscribed to multiple lists, it is difficult to know how many participants are involved. The largest list has over 800 subscribers, so it's safe to assume that there are at least 1,000 subscribers in all. There's a mailing list in this group for just about everyone. The *original scoliosis mailing list* allows discussion of anything to do with scoliosis. There is discussion of both alternative and traditional treatment of scoliosis. The *medical* list does not allow discussion of alternative treatments. The *teen* list is for teen to teen discussion of scoliosis. The *parent* list is for parents to talk to other parents. The *child* list is for discussion of scoliosis in very young children. Finally, all the lists contribute to what is known as the scoliosis digest. The *digest* is normally distributed once a day and contains all e-mails from all of the other five lists. Those participants who want to limit the amount of e-mail they receive will wisely choose the digest.

The Internet Scoliosis Club Forum
www.delphi.com/scolioforum/start/
This is the most active of the bulletin board chat formats. Although there is no indication as to the number of subscribers, there have been over

2,000 messages posted. Most people find it difficult to understand the format during their initial visits. That's obvious from the number of posts that appear in the wrong folders (for example, a discussion on gymnastics appeared in a folder labeled People with Upcoming Surgery). Unfortunately, this site has its share of alternative providers who post advertisements that are thinly disguised as help.

SCOLIOSIS SURGEONS

Not wanting to miss out on the opportunity, a lot of scoliosis surgeons are jumping on the bandwagon with Internet sites of their own. These sites range from single-page sites with the surgeon's contact information to elaborate sites with lots of information.

To find surgeons' Web sites, you could start at www.scoliosis-world.com and click on the link for surgeons that specialize in scoliosis. Or you could contact the Scoliosis Research Society site (see page 167), where you will find names of doctors grouped by state.

ALTERNATIVE CARE

There is no shortage of alternative providers of scoliosis products and "cures" on the Internet. From chiropractors to brace makers, from purveyors of essential oils, nutritional supplements, and even psychic healing, alternative treatment Internet sites vary from amusing (http://abelov.alter-med.cz/) to totally outrageous. There seems to be a never-ending supply of sites that brag about treatments that can prevent progression or even reduce scoliosis curves, despite the lack of any scientific evidence for such claims.

If you have questions about types of treatment being advertised on the Net, you may wish to check out www.Quackwatch.com. It's a fascinating place to go, and if you find a doctor's name there—or a particular technique that sounds suspicious—you should do more research before deciding to try that treatment or to use that doctor.

Research

One can find abstracts of scientific papers by searching Medline. Although they all access the same database, there are dozens of unique Medline search engines on the Internet. One of the best is MedlinePlus (www.medlineplus.org) from the National Institutes of Health. For example, if you wanted to find published papers on the effects of smoking on bone fusion, a search of "smoking and fusion" would turn up about 100 different articles. Although most of the full articles are not available to nonsubscribers, the abstracts that are available often provide enough information for most patients.

For patients interested in the genetics of scoliosis, the Philip Zorab Symposium site at www.ndos.ox.ac.uk/pzs/ has the full text of some interesting papers.

Patient Stories

A rapidly growing number of individuals have posted their scoliosis stories on the Internet. You can find any number of success stories, along with a small number of horror stories. One way to access patient stories is to go to www.scoliosis-world.com and then click on Patient Homepages.

A Last Word

Whether you search for medical information the old fashioned way via magazines, books, and television—or on the information highway via the Internet—you should be aware of how to evaluate medical information. Always remind yourself that just because it's in print doesn't mean it's true. That reminder, however, isn't enough. You should be armed with techniques to help you determine the validity of what you read. In a recent article titled "Medical Propaganda: Whom Do You Believe?" Dr. Robert

Winter, an orthopedic surgeon in Minneapolis, addressed this topic. The following is based on excerpts from that article (reprinted with the permission of The Scoliosis Association).

Patients (and their parents) are bombarded these days with information about medical problems. Television commercials constantly tell us what medication is best—all we have to do is call our doctor and tell him or her to write us a prescription. I'm very glad I'm not a primary care physician having to answer all these calls.

We also have bookstores with endless shelves of books on every conceivable disease or disorder, and to that we have added the Internet, an even more uncontrolled pathway to medical information. Some of it is good, some mediocre, and some downright awful.

How is anyone able to sort through all of this stuff? How do you know what's good and what's not? Whom do you believe?

The answer lies in the scientific method, which, when applied to the medical field, is called "evidence-based medicine." Simply stated, a doctor does not provide a treatment to a patient unless it has been proven to be effective. The main issue, therefore, resolves around the definition of "what is proof?"

Let me begin with a simple example, bacterial pneumonia. Up until the late 1930s, this was commonly a fatal disease. When antibiotics were discovered, the death rate plummeted. This was concrete proof that antibiotics were effective.

Fifteen years ago there was doubt about the effectiveness of bracing for adolescent idiopathic scoliosis. Several well-done scientific studies were performed that proved, with high statistical certainty, that bracing was effective in altering the natural history of the problem. At the same time, these studies showed, with equal statistical validity, that electrical stimulation of the back muscles was absolutely useless. In contrast to these studies, there are no scientific studies that show chiropractic treatment to have any value at all for idiopathic scoliosis.

One of the time-honored methods of influencing people about something medical is the testimonial. This person, whether famous or not, states: "Medicine X is wonderful. It worked for me." This is something we see constantly on TV, and it is absolutely without value. Testimonials can also be negative, as in the now-famous 20/20 television show in which people talked about their terrible troubles "caused by" pedicle screws. In reality, pedicle screws have been a great advance in spine surgery, well proven by the scientific method, and approved by the FDA.

We constantly see new spinal devices, either braces or implants, being advertised or promoted. Quite often these promotions are done without any scientific evidence at all, but sometimes there is a bit of "pseudoscience" thrown in. An example of pseudoscience would be a statement such as "Dr. Z. in Berlin has found this device to be highly effective." When tracked down to the source, it turns out that Dr. Z. merely made that comment at some medical congress without any scientific evidence to back it up.

Another bit of pseudoscience is the "preliminary report." In this, the doctor gives some nice-sounding statistics, but in reality the treatment has not reached its logical end point. Any results of spine fusion at six months post surgery are meaningless. Any reports of brace "results" while the patient is still in the brace are equally meaningless.

Yet another form of pseudoscience is in the misuse of statistics, and there are lots of ways for statistics to be misused. One way is to just use those parts of the statistics that support your claim and exclude those that don't. Recently, a certain spine implant was touted as giving "100 percent more stabilization than the intact, normal spine." It sounded great, but in reality the new implant gave less stabilization than pedicle screw fixation and, when combined with pedicle screws, gave 600 percent more stabilization than the intact, normal spine. All of this data was in the scientific study, but not all of it was mentioned in the promotions.

The final comment has to do with what we call controls. A few years ago we did a study of low back pain in patients who had had a scoliosis fusion down to the fourth lumbar vertebra. When examined fifteen years later, almost 40 percent said they had low back pain. This sounded bad, but when we went out into the general population and found an equal number of people of the same sex, same age, same weight, and same activity level, almost 40 percent of them also had low back pain. Therefore, the conclusion of our study was that fusion down to the fourth lumbar vertebra does not make people different from the general population in regard to back pain.

Studies without controls are highly suspect, but we must remember the first example of this article, the benefits of antibiotics for bacterial pneumonia. We cannot deny treatment to someone and potentially cause them harm.

In conclusion, do not fall for testimonials. Do not fall for pseudo-science. Ask your orthopedic spine surgeon what has been proven to work. It's our job as doctors to sort through all of the evidence to seek the truth. You can educate yourself on the Internet, but you can never get the final answer for your individual problem.

Appendix A:
The Spine Patient's Guide

In their respective roles, both patients and doctors have obligations and responsibilities. The following Spine Patient's Guide has been prepared by the International Federation of Scoliosis Associations (IFOSA) to assist patients and their families, as well as the professionals treating them, to fully understand the responsibilities of each to the other.

The Guide has been primarily designed for patients being treated for scoliosis and kyphosis and other related spinal disorders, but can apply in any case involving medical treatment.

The International Federation of Scoliosis Associations recognizes the fact that there are differences in customs and practices affecting the delivery of medical services in the various countries of the world, but these guidelines have been drawn broad enough to be adaptable for use almost everywhere with little or no modifications necessary.

It is the hope of IFOSA that the adoption of these guidelines will enable patients to become more knowledgeable about their medical problems and their possible outcome, and therefore to be more compliant patients during their treatment.

The Patient is entitled to:

1. Receive complete information and guidance from health-care professionals about the diagnosis and optimal course of action, and to discuss the benefits, risks, and costs of appropriate treatment alternatives.
2. Receive all the information necessary, including the expected medical charges, if any, for the patient to give "informed consent" for any proposed procedure or treatment and to make decisions regarding the health care that is recommended by the professional.
3. Seek independent professional (second) opinions. Copies or summaries of medical records including radiographs should be available.
4. Accept or refuse any recommended treatment, and to be told what effect this refusal may have on the patient's physical and emotional health.
5. Confidentiality. The physician should not (unless required and as permitted by law) reveal confidential communications or information without the consent of the patient, even to members of the patient's family.
6. Continuity of health care as long as such care is required.
7. Courtesy, respect, dignity, responsiveness, and timely attention to the patient's needs.

The Patient should:

1. Inform the physician of his or her comprehensive medical history and all current medical problems.
2. Following informed consent, be compliant and cooperative with the treatment plan that has been proposed by the professional and accepted by the patient.

The Professional is entitled to:

1. Receive full disclosure from the patient of his or her comprehensive medical history and all current medical problems and disclosure as

to whether the patient is seeking medical advice or treatment from another source at the same time.

2. Expect compliance and cooperation on the part of the patient and his or her family.
3. Be advised by the patient if they are not, cannot, or will not follow the recommended course of treatment, so that the professional will be able to properly evaluate the results of treatment.
4. Discharge a patient who is continually uncooperative or non-compliant with the treatment plan.

The Professional should:

1. Request a comprehensive and current medical history of the patient.
2. Give sufficient information to the patient to make an informed decision at each stage of treatment and to advise the patient what effect refusal of treatment may have on the patient's physical and emotional health.
3. Provide continuity of treatment as required as long as the patient is compliant with the treatment plan, unless the professional has given the patient sufficient opportunity to make alternative arrangements.
4. Serve as the patient's advocate by fostering the patient's rights and advise the patient of his or her rights, as stated in this document, even if the patient does not ask for any information.

Appendix B:
Recommended Reading

NATIONAL SCOLIOSIS FOUNDATION RESOURCES

The following is a list of resources that the National Scoliosis Foundation (NSF) recommends for parents and young people. Orders should be sent to the National Scoliosis Foundation, 5 Cabot Place, Stoughton, MA 02072.

The Brace and *Her Brace Is No Handicap*. An illustrated short story and a true story, each concerning a teenage girl coping successfully with scoliosis. *The Brace* was written by Mary Langford; *Her Brace Is No Handicap* was written by Carolyn Callison. Both are reprints from *Young Miss* magazine. Write to NSF and include $1.00 for a single copy.

Getting a Second Opinion. A reprint from *Health Tips*, a publication of the California Medical Education and Research Foundation. For a single copy, send a self-addressed, stamped (first-class stamp), business-size envelope to NSF.

NSF General Packet. A packet containing general information on scoliosis. Write to NSF for details.

NSF Adult Packet. A packet containing information of interest to adults with scoliosis. Write to NSF for details.

1 in Every 10 Persons Has Scoliosis. A brochure that explains what scoliosis is and how to screen for it. It also contains facts about NSF. For a single copy, send a self-addressed, stamped (first-class stamp), business-size envelope. Specify English or Spanish version when writing to NSF.

Reprints of *Medical Update* column from *The Spinal Connection.* Reprints are available on the following topics: adult scoliosis; scoliosis and pregnancy; answers to questions about mild curves: electrical stimulation; Cotrel-Dubousset technique; x-rays; and understanding medical terminology. Send a self-addressed, stamped (first-class stamp), business-size envelope to NSF and specify topic of interest.

Scoliosis . . . Now it can be treated in adults as well as children. A reprint from *Cleveland Magazine.* For a single copy, send a self-addressed, stamped (first-class stamp), business-size envelope to NSF.

A Scoliosis Patient Becomes a Model. A reprint from *Children's Today,* a publication of The Children's Hospital, Boston. For a single copy send a self-addressed, stamped (first-class stamp), business-size envelope to NSF.

The Spinal Connection. A newsletter published by NSF in the spring and fall. It is full of interesting articles concerning the foundation, plus a *Medical Update* column that discusses facts about scoliosis. Contact NSF for subscription information.

Straightened Back, Strengthened Character. Written by Paul Dienhart, a reprint from the Summer 1983 issue of *Health Sciences,* a publication of the University of Minnesota. For a single copy, send a self-addressed, stamped (first-class stamp), business-size envelope to NSF.

The Treatment of Spinal Curvature. Written by Kathleen Doheny, an in-depth article for the layperson concerning current treatment for abnormal spinal curvature. First printed in January 1987. Send a self-addressed, stamped (first-class stamp), business-size envelope along with $1.00 to NSF.

OTHER RESOURCES

The following pamphlets may also be helpful. Note that all orders must be prepaid in United States currency and mailed to the addresses listed below.

Adult Scoliosis Surgery . . . It Can Be Done. A booklet describing various types of surgery for the adult scoliosis patient. Covers the two-stage spine fusion, halo-traction, and other techniques. $4.50 for a single copy. Order from St. Luke's Spine Center, 11311 Shaker Boulevard, Cleveland, OH 44104.

Adult Spinal Deformity. A basic handbook for adult patients that discusses scoliosis and kyphosis. Send $.50 to the Scoliosis Research Society, P.O. Box 2001, Park Ridge, IL 60068.

The AMA Book of Back Care. A book of information on back care compiled in 1982 by the American Medical Association. Cost is $12.95. Write Random House, 201 East 50th Street, New York, NY 10022.

Backtalk. A newsletter for parents and young people. Write the Scoliosis Association, Inc., P.O. Box 51353, Raleigh, NC 27609 for information on subscription rates.

Brace Yourself. Third edition, $3.00 each (100 or more, $2.50 each). Write St. Luke's Spine Center, 11311 Shaker Boulevard, Cleveland, OH 44104.

Going Home. Instructions for pediatric and adult patients who have had a spinal fusion. Includes fourteen inserts to choose from in order to meet the patient's individual needs. $2.50 each. Write the University Hospital Spine Center, 2074 Abington Road, Cleveland, OH 44106 for a list of inserts.

Reducing Patient Exposure During Scoliosis Radiology. Available cost-free from the Food and Drug Administration. Write FDA/HFZ, Rockville, MD 20857 and ask for Order Number FDA 85-8252.

Scoliosis. A brochure describing the cause, prevention, and treatment of scoliosis, kyphosis, and lordosis. Write for details concerning cost to the American Academy of Orthopaedic Surgeons, P.O. Box 618, Park Ridge, IL 60068.

Scoliosis—A Handbook for Patients. Offers information on the detection and treatment of adolescent and adult scoliosis, kyphosis, and lordosis. $1.50 each. Write the Scoliosis Research Society, P.O. Box 2001, Park Ridge, IL 60068.

Scoliosis and Kyphosis. Provides information and advice for the parents of scoliosis patients. $.50 each. Write the Scoliosis Research Society, P.O. Box 2001, Park Ridge, IL 60068.

Scoliosis! Me? An illustrated pamphlet by Dr. Richard A. Marks that gives detailed answers to questions most asked by patients. Cost is $2.50 each. Write to the North Dallas Scoliosis Center, 1910 North Collins Boulevard, Richardson, TX 75080.

Scoliosis Road Map. Written for teenagers, the pamphlet unfolds to a 22-inch by 23-inch poster. $1.50 each. Write the University Hospital Spine Center, 2074 Abington Road, Cleveland, OH 44106.

Scoliosis Surgery: What's It All About? The pamphlet answers many of the questions patients ask before having surgery. $.75 each. Write the University Hospital Spine Center, 2074 Abington Road, Cleveland, OH 44106.

What If You Need an Operation for Scoliosis? Third edition, $3.00 each (100 or more, $2.50 each). Write St. Luke's Spine Center, 11311 Shaker Boulevard, Cleveland, OH 44104.

What Young People and Their Parents Need to Know About Scoliosis. Information from a physical therapist's perspective. $1.00 for a single copy. (50 copies for $34.50 requires prepayment and a $2.00 shipping and handling cost.) Write the American Physical Therapy Association, 1111 No. Fairfax Street, Alexandria, VA 22314.

When the Spine Curves. Available cost-free from the Food and Drug Administration. Write FDA/HFZ, Rockville, MD 20857 and ask for Order Number FDA 85-4198.

You and Your Brace. $.75 each. Write the University Hospital Spine Center, 2074 Abington Road, Cleveland, OH 44106.

Appendix C:

Resources

ORGANIZATIONS

National Scoliosis Foundation, Inc.
5 Cabot Place
Stoughton, MA 02072
800–NSF–MYBACK, 800–673–6922 or 781–341–6333
Fax: 781–341–8333
www.scoliosis.org

*Founded in 1976, the National Scoliosis Foundation (NSF) is a nonprofit or-
ganization devoted to alerting the public to the potentially serious health
problems associated with abnormal spinal curvatures, and to promoting early
detection and timely preventive professional treatment through the screening
of every child aged ten to fifteen, the critical growth years.*

*To reach its goal of eliminating the effects of abnormal progressive spinal
curvatures, the staff and volunteers of NSF maintain a resource center; work
in close cooperation with writers, publishers, and producers; make presen-*

tations to appropriate groups; and provide easy-to-read literature for individuals, health centers, schools, and spine clinics. In addition, they are consultants for people interested in required school screenings and have testified before legislative committees when invited. NSF also publishes a biannual newsletter, The Spinal Connection, and provides information on guidelines and materials for implementing and improving screening programs with follow-up for parents. The foundation has produced an educational unit on scoliosis for the prescreening education of students in fifth through seventh grades. This includes an audiovisual presentation, teacher's guide, poster, brochure, and resource sheets listing sources for additional materials. For more information, write to NSF at the above address.

The Scoliosis Association, Inc.
P.O. Box 811705
Boca Raton, FL 33481-1705
800–800–0669
Fax: 407–368–8518

Founded in 1976 by the parents of scoliosis patients, the Scoliosis Association is a nonprofit organization. It has among its goals educating the general public about scoliosis and other spinal deviations. It also encourages and sponsors scoliosis screening programs. To obtain information on the publications, films, and tapes available, write to the association directly.

The Scoliosis Association publishes a newsletter, Backtalk, four times a year. All members of the chapters and the association receive this newsletter, which prints news likely to be of interest to scoliosis patients and others in medical and educational fields. For information about membership applications and dues, write to the association.

The association also sponsors the formation of scoliosis chapters throughout the country. These chapters are parent/patient support groups that afford the scoliosis patient and his or her family a meeting place every month with other families involved with scoliosis. At these meetings, members can help one another to effect a positive social and emotional adjustment during the treatment of scoliosis. To find out if there is a support group in your area, call or write the headquarters of the Scoliosis Association at the above address.

Scoliosis Research Society
611 East Wells Street
Milwaukee, WI 53202
414–289–9107
Fax: 414–276–3349
www.srs.org

Founded in 1966, the Scoliosis Research Society (SRS) is a nonprofit organization composed of orthopedic surgeons and spine specialists who are dedicated to education, research, and treatment of spinal deformities. The SRS also sponsors an annual meeting that is a forum for the presentation of the most current research results. The organization is an affiliate of the American Academy of Orthopaedic Surgeons, and it publishes a number of informative materials on scoliosis. For more information about available publications and films, write to the SRS.

American Academy of Orthopaedic Surgeons
6300 North River Road
Rosemont, IL 60018-4226
708–346–2267
Fax: 708–823–8026
www.aaos.org

The American Academy of Orthopaedic Surgeons (AAOS) is a not-for-profit organization founded in 1933. AAOS is the largest medical organization for musculoskeletal specialists. Members of the academy have completed medical school and up to five years of specialty study in orthopedics in an accredited residency program, passed a comprehensive oral and written exam, and have been certified by the American Board of Orthopaedic Surgery.

AAOS is committed to increasing the public's awareness of musculoskeletal conditions such as scoliosis, with an emphasis on preventive measures. For more information about available AAOS publications, contact their communications and publications department.

Products

Orthotic Undergarment Company
Route 6, Box 46-H
Austin, Texas 78737

Custom-made undergarments to wear under scoliosis braces.

Brace Mates
P.O. Box 200
Concord, VA 24538

Custom-made undergarments to wear under scoliosis braces.

Index

Page numbers in italics refer to illustrations.